Medicines Management in Children's Nursing

Karen Blair

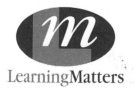

LearningMatters

First published in 2011 by Learning Matters Ltd

British Library Cataloguing in Publication Data
A CIP record for this book is available from the British Library

ISBN: 978 1 84445 470 9

This book is also available in the following ebook formats:

Adobe ebook: 978 1 84445 753 3
ePub ebook: 978 1 84445 752 6
Kindle: 978 0 85725 017 9

Cover and text design by Toucan Design
Project Management by Diana Chambers
Typeset by Kelly Winter
Printed and bound in Great Britain by Short Run Press Ltd, Exeter, Devon

Learning Matters Ltd
20 Cathedral Yard
Exeter EX1 1HB
Tel: 01392 215560
E-mail: info@learningmatters.co.uk
www.learningmatters.co.uk

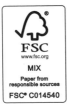

FSC
www.fsc.org
MIX
Paper from
responsible sources
FSC® C014540

Contents

Foreword

The management and administration of medicines is a key aspect of nursing practice and is one of the most common therapeutic interventions in healthcare. Administering medications to children requires very specific knowledge and understanding. To safely and effectively prepare medications for children, special consideration has to be given to accurate dosages, the developmental stages of children, and working in partnership with parents, carers and the children themselves. This text provides an excellent assistant to the children's nursing student undertaking a pre-registration programme and a reference for qualified staff to ensure confidence in administering medicines in their practice.

The text is thorough and clearly written, beginning with a review of your calculation skills, which can then send you off on a path to deeper understanding of the complexities of pharmacological knowledge, managing conditions, establishing good practice, and learning the fundamental techniques of medication administration and storage.

The author has included a wider view of medicines management in children's nursing, covering ethical and legal issues, working with other professionals, health promotion and lifestyle advice, and working in both hospital and community settings. There is also a section on complementary and alternative uses of medicines. In the final chapter the evidence for practising safe medicines management is explored through research to underpin clinical judgement and evidenced-based practice. There are many activities and examples to help you embed the knowledge into your practice and encourage you on a path of lifelong learning as an up-to-date practitioner.

Dr Shirley Bach
Series Editor

About the author

Karen Blair was a Senior Lecturer in Children's Nursing at Canterbury Christ Church University while writing this book. She has remained an honorary lecturer at Canterbury since taking up her present post as a nurse practitioner in General Practice in Norwich. She has worked in a wide range of children's services since 1987, in both acute and community, the latter as a health visitor, nurse prescriber and nurse practitioner. She has an MSc in Advanced Paediatric Ambulatory Care, and worked in the UK's first Children's Walk-in-Centre in Liverpool before becoming a lecturer at Canterbury.

Introduction

The purpose of this book is to introduce child nursing students and other interested nurses to the management of medicines in children and young people. The administration of medicines forms a significant part of almost every nurse's everyday practice and is the most common intervention carried out in the NHS. It is hoped that the contents of this book will provide you with the knowledge required to meet the standards of competency for safe practice in the management and administration of medicines to children and young people.

Why 'Medicines Management in Children's Nursing'?

Children and young people are different from adults in many ways. Specific knowledge and skills different from those in adult nursing are required by children's nurses in order to provide safe and effective care. It is therefore entirely appropriate that there is a book specifically written on medicines management to meet the needs of nurses who care for children.

Book structure

Chapter 1 introduces you to calculating paediatric drug doses. It is essential that you demonstrate competence in basic medicines calculations by the first progression point of your nurse training. Errors in administration of medicines to children are common and are often due to mistakes being made in calculating drug doses. The chapter starts with basic numeracy skills by reviewing the metric system and simple medicine calculations. It builds on your knowledge to enable you to calculate the more difficult medicine doses sometimes required.

Chapter 2 is about the legal and ethical issues in children's medicines management. This is an important chapter as you must always act within the law in both your professional practice and personal life, as specified in *The Code: Standards of conduct, performance and ethics for nurses and midwives* (NMC, 2008). The law in relation to medicines and consent to treatment is complicated in the UK. This chapter should make you aware of the important legal and ethical principles that will affect your practice.

Chapter 3 is about holistic care and treatment options. The chapter aims to make you aware of the importance of using a holistic approach to the management and care of children/young people and their families. It will increase your awareness of therapies that are complementary and alternative to the use of medicines.

Chapter 4 aims to increase your knowledge of medicines and their actions. The chapter discusses the developmental differences between infants and young children, and between children and adults, which alter the effectiveness of drugs compared to adults. As a nurse you need to understand why it is important to take the child's developmental stage into consideration when administering medications.

Chapter 5 is concerned with the rules governing the storage, ordering and receiving of drugs, of which all nurses need to be aware in order to practise within the law. This chapter addresses such specific issues as storage of controlled drugs and oxygen in hospital and community settings.

Chapter 6 describes the different routes and methods used for the administration of medicines to children. How to use a prescription chart correctly and how to prepare and administer medicines safely and effectively via different routes are fundamental everyday skills of the registered nurse. The chapter also describes how to recognise and manage anaphylaxis.

Chapter 7 is about working in partnership with parents, carers and children. The chapter explores how we can support children, young people and their parents/carers to make safe and informed choices about their medicines.

Chapter 8 is the final chapter and is focused on keeping up to date with evidence-based practice. All nurses must make an effort to keep up to date with practice and provide the highest standard of care based on the best available evidence. This chapter guides you towards the many sources of evidence available to you in order to stay informed and make good decisions about medicines management.

Requirements for the NMC *Standards for Pre-registration Nursing Education* and Essential Skills Clusters

The Nursing and Midwifery Council (NMC) has established standards of competence to be met by applicants to different parts of the register, and these are the standards it considers necessary for safe and effective practice. In addition to the competencies, the NMC has set out specific skills that nursing students must be able to perform at various points of an education programme. These are known as Essential Skills Clusters (ESCs). This book is structured so that it will help you to understand and meet the relevant competencies and ESCs required for entry to the NMC register. The relevant competencies and ESCs are presented at the start of each chapter so that you can clearly see which ones the chapter addresses. There are *generic standards* that all nursing students, irrespective of their field, must achieve, and *field-specific standards* relating to each field of nursing, that is, mental health, children's, learning disability and adult nursing. Most chapters of this book start with the generic standards, followed by the field-specific standards for children's nurses.

This book includes the latest standards for 2010 onwards, taken from the *Standards for Pre-registration Nursing Education* (NMC, 2010a). For links to the pre-2010 standards, please visit the website for the book at **www.learningmatters.co.uk/nursing**.

Learning features

Activities

Throughout the book you will find activities in the text that will help you to make sense of, and learn about, the material being presented by the author. Some activities ask you to reflect on aspects of practice, or your experience of it, or the people or situations you encounter. *Reflection* is an essential skill in nursing, and it helps you to understand the world around you and often to identify how things might be improved. Other activities will help you develop key skills such as your ability to *think critically* about a topic in order to challenge received wisdom, or your ability to *research a topic and find appropriate information and evidence*, and to be able to make decisions using that evidence in situations that are often difficult and time-pressured. Finally, communication and working as part of a team are core to all nursing practice, and some activities will ask you to carry out *group activities* or think about your *communication skills* to help develop these.

All the activities require you to take a break from reading the text, think through the issues presented and carry out some independent study, possibly using the internet. Where appropriate, there are sample answers presented at the end of each chapter, and these will help you to understand more fully your own reflections and independent study. Remember, academic study will always require independent work; attending lectures will never be enough to be successful on your programme, and these activities will help to deepen your knowledge and understanding of the issues under scrutiny and give you practice at working on your own.

You might want to think about completing these activities as part of your personal development plan (PDP) or portfolio. After completing the activity, write it up in your PDP or portfolio in a section devoted to that particular skill, then look back over time to see how far you have developed. You can also do more of the activities for a key skill that you have identified a weakness in, which will help build your skill and confidence in this area.

Glossary

In each chapter you will see a selection of words and terms highlighted in bold print where they first occur in the book. Definitions of these can be found in the Glossary on pages 203–6. For further explanation of unfamiliar terms, see the Glossary on the website for the companion volume, *Introduction to Medicines Management in Nursing*.

Medicines Management series

This book is part of a mini-series. Other titles in this series include:

Introduction to Medicines Management in Nursing, Martina O'Brien, Alison Spires and Kirsty Andrews

Medicines Management in Adult Nursing, Elizabeth Lawson and Dawn L. Hennefer

Medicines Management in Mental Health Nursing, Stanley Mutsatsa

Chapter 1
Calculating children's medicines

Case study

Many years ago, as a fairly newly qualified children's nurse on night duty, I was dealing with a seriously ill baby admitted with meningitis and was supporting a consultant paediatrician and a doctor who was relatively inexperienced in paediatrics. The consultant asked me to prepare the intravenous antibiotics, but the less experienced doctor insisted he would do this himself and did not require my help. The drugs were prepared and administered to the baby by the less experienced doctor swiftly, as the situation warranted, without checking with me or the consultant. As soon as the baby was stabilised, I started tidying up the treatment area, including the drugs used, and picked up an empty gentamicin vial and asked the doctor where it had all gone. He immediately realised his error, as he had mistakenly administered the whole vial to the baby, which was four times the recommended dose. Thankfully the baby recovered, but needed very close monitoring for drug toxicity, which could lead to kidney damage and hearing loss.

Introduction

The above case study highlights the important factors children's nurses should be aware of when calculating and administering medicines to children. Unlike for most adult patients, children's doses need to be calculated on an individual basis according to their age, weight or body surface area. A drug miscalculation in a child can have catastrophic effects and all care needs to be taken to avoid this. As a children's nurse you must have an awareness of what a sensible dose would be for the children in your care, and guide other professionals and parents. You need to be confident and skilled in your ability to calculate doses in all situations.

This chapter will start by reviewing the metric system in order that you are able to understand the basic units of measurement used in the prescribing of drugs and how drug strengths are expressed, including percentages and units. You should feel comfortable about converting from one unit of measurement to another, and understand the terms of expression in medicines. As most drugs are prescribed according to a child's weight, converting weights from imperial to metric will be covered and vice versa, including methods of estimating a child's weight in an emergency situation. This will help you always to have in mind what is a sensible estimate of weight at different ages, so you can be confident the recorded weight on the child's drug chart is correct.

The chapter covers the calculation of tablets and capsules, and the more commonly used liquid medicines and intravenous fluids, and how to work out if the prescribed dose or rate is correct for the child. It is essential that the children's nurse administering the dose is capable of checking the calculation and has an awareness of what a reasonable dose would be. Throughout the chapter there will be worked examples in order to demonstrate the methods used and activities for you to practise the skills needed to gain competence.

The metric system

In order to calculate medicine dosages safely, it is essential to have a clear understanding of the units of measurements used in the prescribing and dispensing of drugs. The strength of medicines should always be expressed using the standard metric system of weights and measures. The basic units used in clinical practice derive from the Système International (SI). The SI units for weight (mass) are shown in Table 1.1 and those for volume in Table 1.2.

Note that nanograms and picograms are rarely used in clinical practice.

The terms 'micrograms', 'nanograms' and 'picograms' should NOT be abbreviated but always written in full. This is to prevent medication error attributable to abbreviations. Abbreviating

Unit	Abbreviation	Equivalent	Abbreviation
1 kilogram	kg	1000 grams	g
1 gram	g	1000 milligrams	mg
1 milligram	mg	1000 micrograms	do not abbreviate
1 microgram	do not abbreviate	1000 nanograms	do not abbreviate
1 nanogram	do not abbreviate	1000 picograms	do not abbreviate

Table 1.1: The SI units for weight (mass)

Unit	Abbreviation	Equivalent	Abbreviation
1 litre	L	1000 millilitres	mL or ml
1 millilitre	mL or ml	1000 microlitres	do not abbreviate

Table 1.2: The SI units for volume

micrograms as μg (the official abbreviation for microgram in the SI system) can be mistaken for mg and lead to a one thousandfold dosage error.

Note that the term 'millilitre' (ml or mL) is used in medicine and pharmacy rather than cubic centimetre abbreviated as 'cc', as this can be mistaken for 'u' (units) when poorly written.

The term 'litre' is generally not abbreviated to avoid error. It is safer to express volume in millilitres in order to avoid the unnecessary use of decimal points, which can lead to dosage errors.

You must be able to differentiate between the units of measurement and convert one unit into another. Getting the decimal point in the right place when converting from grams to milligrams and to micrograms is essential.

You should be able to see that the relationship between the units is in multiples of 1000. Drugs may be prescribed for children in grams, milligrams, micrograms and sometimes nanograms. You need to be able to recognise different units and be able to change one unit to another. In order to change from one unit to another, you need to move your decimal point to the left or right in order to divide or multiply by 1000.

Worked example

When converting grams to mgs or vice versa the decimal point moves three places:

5g = 5000mg
0.5g = 500mg
0.05g = 50mg
0.005g = 5mg.

When converting milligrams to micrograms the decimal point moves three places:

5mg = 5000 micrograms
50mg = 50,000 micrograms
500mg = 500,000 micrograms.

continued opposite . . .

continued . . . .

When converting micrograms to nanograms the decimal point moves three places:

5 micrograms = 5000 nanograms
50 micrograms = 50,000 nanograms
500 micrograms = 500,000 nanograms.

When converting litres to millilitres the decimal point moves three places:

5 litres = 5000 millilitres (mL)
5000 millilitres = 5,000,000 microlitres.

Some important points to remember in order to avoid errors by misreading are as follows.

- Take great care when placing your decimal points in order to avoid tenfold drug errors.
- The unnecessary use of decimal points should be avoided, for example write 5mg, not 5.0mg.
- Always write a zero before a decimal point for numbers less than 1, for example write '0.3', never '.3'.
- When working in fractions of a milligram, use micrograms to avoid error. For example, 0.3mg would be written as 300 micrograms.
- Abbreviations are always singular, for example 'mg' not 'mgs'.

Now try the following conversion exercises.

Activity 1.1

Convert the following measurements. You may find the table below useful.

1										grams (g)
1	0	0	0							milligrams (mg)
1	0	0	0	0	0	0				micrograms
1	0	0	0	0	0	0	0	0	0	nanograms

continued overleaf . . .

continued . . .

1. 250 micrograms into milligrams
2. 1345 milligrams into micrograms
3. 3000 nanograms into micrograms
4. 1.34 kilograms into grams
5. 145g into kilograms
6. 0.07g into milligrams
7. 0.45 micrograms into nanograms
8. 500 milligrams into grams

Answers are provided at the end of the chapter.

The above activity should enable you to convert one SI unit of weight to another. Continue to practise this until you feel you are fully proficient at doing so. If you are having difficulty with these conversions, you must seek out further help and advice. Remember – never administer a drug dose unless you are absolutely confident in your calculation.

Activity 1.2

Convert the following volumes:

1. 500mL into L
2. 1.2L into mL
3. 30mL into microlitres
4. 6000 microlitres into mL

Answers are provided at the end of the chapter.

The above activity should enable you to convert one SI unit of volume to another. Remember – when converting litres to millilitres you need to times by 1000, or the decimal point moves three places to the right. When converting millilitres to litres you need to divide by 1000, or the decimal point moves three places to the left.

A recurring theme in drug errors involving children concerns errors of calculation (NPSA, 2007). A misplaced decimal point can mean a tenfold drug overdose or underdose. Mistakes in converting one unit to another have had catastrophic consequences in the past for children, in particular for neonates, where drug doses are very small and a misplaced decimal point would make a substantial error.

Case studies

In 1996 a 6-week-old baby was admitted to intensive care at Treliske Hospital, Truro, after being administered ten times the prescribed amount of morphine. He stopped breathing and needed resuscitating and suffered severe fits. The hospital admitted he was given 4mg of morphine instead of 0.4mg following a routine hernia operation (Jury, 1996).

Newborn twins were treated with intramuscular gentamicin for suspected septicaemia. It was realised after two doses that the infants had received 50mg per dose instead of 5mg due to a nurse misreading the prescription. The twins developed acute renal failure, but fortunately gradually improved over several weeks (Koren et al., 1986).

One-day-old, 1.5kg premature baby Louise Wood died an hour after a hospital doctor gave her 100 times the safe amount of morphine at Rotherham District General Hospital in 1995. The dose was drawn up by a junior doctor, who made a calculation error and placed a decimal point in the wrong place. The dosage should have been checked before it was administered but it was not (Dyer, 1999).

The above cases highlight how essential accuracy is when calculating drug doses for infants, and how important it is that nurses have the ability to check what a reasonable dose for a child's weight is. Most drug doses in children are calculated according to their weight in kilograms and this will be discussed later in this chapter.

Units of activity

For some medicines the strength of the drug is expressed in units of activity per given volume rather than using metric units. This is usually the case for medicines produced from natural sources such as insulin, hormones and vitamins. These products are standardised using biological assays and their strength is expressed in units. For example, insulin is expressed as 100 units/mL, heparin as 1000 units/mL or nystatin as 100 000 units/mL. It is not essential that you know the quantity of the units of activity in relation to the metric system. However, you need to be aware of how to interpret prescriptions for these products.

'Units' should always be written in full and not abbreviated as 'u', which can easily be mistaken for a zero, leading to dosage error.

Measurement of insulin

Insulin should be measured and administered using specially manufactured disposable insulin syringes, and not the standard intravenous syringes. Insulin syringes are specifically calibrated in units of insulin rather than mL, in order to simplify drawing up a measured dose and avoid error. The dilution of different types of insulin (such as soluble insulin, insulin glargine or isophane insulin) is such that 1mL volume of fluid has 100 standard units of that product.

Activity 1.3

Jade is a 3-month-old infant admitted to the ward with oral thrush. She has been prescribed nystatin oral suspension 100,000 units 4 times daily after feeds. Nystan suspension is available as Nystatin 100,000 units/mL.

- How much suspension would you administer for each dose?

An answer is provided at the end of the chapter.

Although the above prescription looks quite complicated, it is a relatively easy calculation to work out.

Weight and body surface area

Most drugs are prescribed to children according to their weight in kilograms. The child should always be weighed as soon as possible, using scales that are calibrated on a regular basis and are suitable for the age of the child. Children under 2 years should be weighed naked, and those over 2 years in minimal clothing (RCN, 2010). The weight should be recorded in kilograms on the appropriate drug chart or patient records. It is policy in some units for two nurses to check the weight, as an error in recording weight could mean the child is prescribed an incorrect dose of medication.

It is useful to have an awareness of what a reasonable weight would be for a child of a particular age. This will help you to identify errors in recordings of weight, to estimate a weight in an emergency situation or identify calculation errors. Length-based estimates are taken using a measurement tape device (such as Broselow Paediatric Emergency Tape), which is a long strip of laminated paper divided into different coloured areas that correspond to patients' height. The tape provides all the information, including drug dosage for emergency resuscitation of a child up to 36kg.

Table 1.3 shows mean values for weight, height and gender by age that can be referred to in the absence of actual measurements; however, it is important to look at children to assess if they are of average weight for their age as this varies considerably. The child's actual weight and height should be obtained as soon as possible and the dose recalculated (BMA et al., 2010).

If a child's age is known and is 1–10 years, the following formula is commonly accepted and used to estimate weight for children:

Weight (kg) = 2 × (age in years + 4).

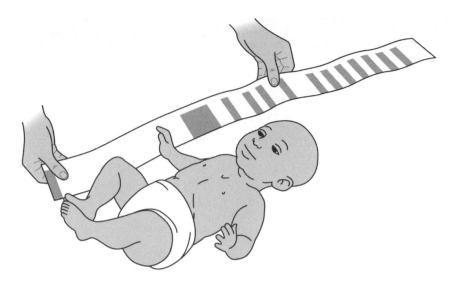

Figure 1.1: Using a Broselow Paediatric Emergency Tape

Age	Weight (kg)	Height (cm)
Full-term neonate	3.5	51
1 month	4.3	55
2 months	5.4	58
3 months	6.1	61
4 months	6.7	63
6 months	7.6	67
1 year	9	75
3 years	14	96
5 years	18	109
7 years	23	122
10 years	32	138
12 years	39	149
14-year-old boy	49	163
14-year-old girl	50	159
Adult male	68	176
Adult female	58	164

Table 1.3: Mean table of weights (BMA et al., 2010)

Worked example

You are working in the accident and emergency department and you receive a call alerting the staff to the arrival of Ben, aged 4 years, in status epilepticus. You need to have some drugs available for the anaesthetist but you need to know his weight.

- weight (Kg) = 2 × (4 years + 4)
- weight (Kg) = 2 × (8)
- estimated weight for Ben = 16Kg

Length-based and age-based estimations of a child's weight are both suitable methods in an emergency. Length-based estimates have been found to be statistically better, but the difficulty in attempting to measure a child during resuscitation may support the simplicity of using the child's age against the growth chart (Sandell and Charman, 2009).

The activity below should familiarise you with using the formula method to estimate a child's weight in an emergency.

Activity 1.4

Using the formula method, estimate the weight of a child aged:

1. 2 years
2. 6 years
3. 10 years
4. 5 years.

Compare your answers with the mean table of weights from the *British National Formulary for Children* (BNFC) (BMA et al., 2010) (Table 1.3 above). Are your answers reasonable?

Answers are provided at the end of the chapter.

Remember that a child's actual weight and height may vary considerably from the table values and the formula method, so it is important to see the child before applying them to check that they are appropriate. As soon as possible the child's actual weight should be measured.

Converting between metric and imperial units

You should always weigh the child in kilograms to obtain an accurate weight, and not rely on a parent's reported weight, which may be wrong or not recent enough to be accurate. However, many parents still feel more comfortable and familiar with the imperial units of pounds and ounces for their child's weight, and you may be asked to convert a child's weight from pounds to kilograms and vice versa. The easiest way to do this would be to refer to a weight conversion chart, which should be readily available in clinics, the ward or sometimes in the Parent Held Child Health Record (PHCHR) or 'Red Book'. If you go online and access the BNFC, go to 'Resources' then 'Calculators' and you will find a useful imperial–metric conversion calculator for weight, length and volume (see the 'Useful website' at the end of this chapter for the web address).

You will find it useful to learn the following conversion values, as parents will expect you to have some understanding of their language of weights and measures.

*   1kg = 2.2 pounds (lb)
*   14lb = 1 stone
*   16 ounces (oz) = 1lb

The following examples demonstrate how to convert imperial measures to metric and vice versa.

Worked example

Converting pounds to kilograms

Reece is reported to weigh 2 stone 12lb by his parents; you want to know how much he weighs in kilograms.

First, you need to change the weight into pounds by multiplying the stones by 14:

2 stone 12lb = (2 x 14) + 12lb = 40lb.

Next, convert the pounds into kg by dividing by 2.2:

40 ÷ 2.2 = 18.18kg.

Converting from kilograms into pounds

You have just weighed Tamara and she weighed 6.5kg. Her parents want to know what this weight is in pounds.

continued overleaf . . .

continued . . .

> First, you need to change Kilograms into pounds by multiplying by 2.2:
>
> 6.5 × 2.2 = 14.3lb.
>
> You need to convert the 0.3lb into ounces:
>
> 1lb = 16oz, so 0.3lb = 0.3 × 16 = 4.8oz.
>
> Therefore, the baby weighs 14lb 5oz (to the nearest ounce).

The activity below will help you practise converting pounds to kilograms and kilograms to pounds.

Activity 1.5

Use the conversion values to convert these weights to the nearest two decimal places.

1. 7lb 12oz into kg
2. 3 stone into kg
3. 1 stone 8lb into kg
4. 3.6kg into lb
5. 24.5kg into lb

Answers are provided at the end of the chapter.

In order to save time on calculations, it is useful to have a weight conversion chart readily available next to the scales for staff and parents to refer to. Parents are very interested in knowing their child's weight, but unless it is in the values they are used to it can be meaningless.

Body surface area estimations

A body surface area (BSA) estimation can be a more accurate indicator than body weight for a child's ability to metabolise a drug. Medicine doses based on BSA are most likely to be used in paediatric oncology and in the use of **cytotoxic** drugs. Many physiological phenomena that influence drug disposition, such as renal and hepatic function and metabolic rate, correlate better with BSA. There are many formulae and nomograms to estimate BSA from height and weight.

Children's nurses are familiar with the difficulties in obtaining accurate height and weight measurements of children and serious errors in determining BSA have been reported. To overcome the significant errors in determining height measurements in children and infants, the Boyd estimates of BSA have been used by the UK Children's Cancer and Leukaemia Group (Sharkey et al., 2001) to construct a table based on weight alone. Tables for BSA based on the Boyd equation can be found inside the back cover of the BNFC.

Calculating children's medicines and forms of medicine

The calculation of drug dosages is an important part of what registered children's nurses do frequently in clinical practice and, in order to do so safely, children's nurses must have key knowledge and skills in this area of practice. It is the nurse's responsibility to check prior to administration of a drug that the dose is correct (NMC, 2004). Recent evidence has highlighted that medication errors are a significant problem in paediatrics (Ghaleb et al., 2006; Walsh et al., 2005). Drug doses for children are calculated individually, and can be according to the child's age, weight, BSA or clinical condition. This leads to the increased potential for dosing errors.

Some healthcare professionals have difficulty in calculating the correct dose (Gladstone, 1995), errors being due to calculation mistakes, misplacement of the decimal point and use of incorrect units, for example milligrams instead of micrograms. Junior doctors who are unfamiliar with paediatric doses and lack experience and training have the potential to make calculation errors also (Sammons and Conroy, 2008; Conroy et al., 2008). It is therefore essential that the nurse administrating the prescribed dose is capable of checking the calculation and has an awareness of what a reasonable dose would be.

Suitable strengths of formulations may not be manufactured for children, as they are designed for adults and are not commercially available for children. This increases the risk for errors in dosage calculation, as complex calculations and dilutions are required to arrive at the appropriate formulation. For example, it may be necessary to use an **ampoule** that contains more than ten times the required dose to draw up an injection for a neonate (Chappell and Newman, 2004; Tan et al., 2003).

Estimation

It is essential that you use your common sense when performing any calculation and have an awareness of what a sensible answer would be. You should develop your skills to be able to estimate what a calculation would be in order to check and review that you have the answer correct. This is particularly important when the calculation involves decimal points.

Worked example

A child is prescribed chloral hydrate 500mg, which you have available as 200mg per 5mL.

5 5 12·5

- Estimate first - do you need more or less of the available dosage?
- Look for a relationship between the numbers involved.
- You should be able to recognise that 500 is 2½ times 200.
- So if there is 200mg in 5mL, there will be 500mg in 2½ × 5ml = 12.5mL.

Worked example

An infant is prescribed flucloxacillin 37.5mg and you have available flucloxacillin syrup 125mg in 5mL.

- You can estimate that flucloxacillin 37.5mg is less than half of the available strength, but slightly more than a quarter.
- A quarter of 125mg/5mL would be a dose of 1.25mL.
- So we know our answer should be slightly more than 1.25mL, but less than half of 5mL, which is 2.5mL.

In order to work out the exact amount

If we do the calculation:

$$\frac{37.5}{125} \times 5 = 1.5\text{mL}$$

continued opposite . . .

continued . . .

we can review our answer with our estimate, and be reassured
that our answer lies within a reasonable amount.

It would be good practice to get into a routine of estimating your answers in this way.

Using a calculator

You should be able to carry out simple and straightforward medicines calculations without the use of a calculator. A calculator will only give the answer to what is keyed in, and it is too easy to press the wrong button and come up with a wrong answer, or get the decimal point in the wrong place. It is acceptable to work out the dose, and then check your answer by using a calculator. When more complex calculations are required, it may be necessary to use a calculator, but you must have an awareness of what a sensible answer would be if you do this. Be sure that you are familiar with your calculator and test yourself using simple calculations that you know the answers to.

Checking the dose

You must also have an awareness of what a reasonable dose would be for each individual child, as you cannot assume that the **prescriber** is correct. You have a responsibility to check the dose before you administer it by referring to the latest edition of the BNFC. If at all unsure, do not administer the drug; inform the prescriber, and ask for help from somebody more experienced. It is the policy of many hospitals for two nurses to check all drugs for children; you should check your local policy and adhere to it. Double-checking drug calculations is thought to be effective in reducing hospital medication errors (Miller et al., 2006). However, having two nurses to check all drug calculations and doses is not always practical, particularly for community children's nurses who often work alone. Some studies (O'Shea, 1999) have demonstrated that single-nurse administration of drugs resulted in fewer errors, whereas other studies have shown that two-nurse administration had fewer mistakes. The evidence seems inconclusive, so you should be guided by local policy.

Activity 1.6   *Reflection*

Think about times where you have been asked to second-check a dosage calculation for a child on the ward.

- How often have you disagreed with the calculation of your colleague?
- What pressures are you under to agree with your colleague?
- What strategies would you use if you both disagreed?
- Do you think single-nurse administration would be more effective and efficient than double-checking?

An outline answer is provided at the end of the chapter.

It is likely that you will be responsible for second-checking drug dosage calculations with a more senior colleague in practice. It is possible that, at times, you may disagree with your senior colleague's calculation and you may feel pressured into agreeing with them. You should always have confidence in your own ability, and if need be ask for a third person, perhaps a doctor or pharmacist, when there is a calculation discrepancy. A literature review (O'Shea, 1999) found that drug calculation performance was not superior in those nurses with years of experience. The nurses with experience tended to be more certain of themselves, despite being wrong in their judgement. It is possible that more errors are made by experienced staff than by those who are more recently qualified.

Tablets and capsules

It is the responsibility of a children's nurse to calculate the correct dose and number of tablets or capsules to be administered to a child. Tablets and capsules are dispensed in the form of a given weight of the drug that has been compounded with other products to make it suitable for administration. Tablets can be dispensed in either a dispersible or effervescent form that must be dissolved in water, or that is designed to dissolve in the mouth, or designed to be chewed.

Calculating tablets

The dosages of tablets and capsules have been manufactured in accordance with commonly prescribed therapeutic doses for adults. For example, a therapeutic dose of paracetamol is 500mg every 4–6 hours. Paracetamol tablets are manufactured as 500mg tablets so that it is easy to administer a therapeutic dose to an adult. Tablets and capsules are less commonly used for children because of the impossibility of administering specific doses for weight, and because younger children may be unable to swallow them.

Some calculations that you may be required to do are so straightforward that you may be able to work them out using mental arithmetic. This is often the case for tablets and capsules.

Worked example

A child is prescribed amoxicillin 250mg, which is available in the form of amoxicillin capsules 250mg. How many capsules should be administered?

This is a straightforward calculation. Both the prescription and the label are in the same units (mg).

The answer is one capsule.

Some calculations are more difficult, and if the answer is not easily obvious to you it would be sensible to use a formula or equation.

Worked example

A child is prescribed 20mg of oral prednisolone, which is available in the form of prednisolone 5mg tablets. How many tablets do you need to administer?

There are different ways to do this and no right or wrong way as long as you come up with the right answer!

You could keep adding the 5mg doses until you reach 20mg.

$$1 \times 5mg = 5mg$$
$$2 \times 5mg = 10mg$$
$$3 \times 5mg = 15mg$$
$$4 \times 5mg = 20mg.$$

It is also possible to use an equation to solve your tablets and capsule dosage calculations and you should become familiar with this:

$$\frac{\text{Dose required (what you want)}}{\text{Strength available (what you have)}}.$$

The dose prescribed, or what you want, is 20mg.
The dose per tablet or what you have got, is 5mg.

$$\frac{20mg}{5mg} = 4$$

The patient will be given 4 tablets.

The following activity will help you to practise using the equation in order to calculate how many tablets to administer for a prescribed dose.

Activity 1.7

Use the equation to calculate correctly the number of tablets or capsules to administer for the following prescriptions.

1. Paracetamol 240mg   Available as paediatric soluble tablets paracetamol 120mg.
2. Sodium valproate 300mg   Available as sodium valproate tablets 100mg.
3. Prednisolone 40mg   Available as prednisolone 5mg tablets.
4. Diazepam 4mg   Available as diazepam 2mg tablets.

Answers are provided at the end of the chapter.

The above calculations have been straightforward, as the prescription and the available tablets have been in the same units. Sometimes the prescription is written in different units from those of the available formulation.

Worked example

Your patient requires 0.5g of flucloxacillin. The capsules available are 250mg. How many capsules would you administer?

First you need to convert your measurements into the same units. The simplest way is to convert into units that will eliminate the decimal point, which will make your calculation easier. This usually involves converting the prescribed dose into the unit used for the capsule weight. In this case we need to convert grams to milligrams.

1g = 1000mg

Therefore, you need to multiply 0.5 x 1000, which equals 500mg.

continued opposite . . .

continued . . . .

Now you need to work out how many grams you need to make up the 500mg dose. There are different ways to do this. The most common is adding the 250mg doses until you reach 500mg.

250mg + 250mg = 500mg.

Or to use the formula:

$$\frac{\text{What you want}}{\text{What you have got}} = \frac{500mg}{250mg} = 2 \text{ capsules}$$

Activity 1.8

Try the following calculations in which the prescriptions are in different units from those of the formulations available.

1. Digoxin 0.25mg   Available as digoxin 250 microgram tablets.
2. Cefradine 1g   Available as cefradine 250mg capsules.
3. Tetracycline 0.5g   Available as tetracycline 250mg tablets.

Answers are provided at the end of the chapter.

Liquid medicines

Liquid medicines are commonly prescribed for children as they have often not developed the ability to swallow tablets and capsules.

Calculating liquid doses

The usual way of denoting a concentration of a liquid medicine is by milligrams of drug per millilitre of liquid. For example, paracetamol is available in 120mg per 5mL or 250mg per 5mL.

If the prescribed dose is straightforward, such as 120mg of paracetamol, the calculation is simple. For more complex calculations we can use a formula:

$$\frac{\text{What you want (strength required)}}{\text{What you have got (strength available)}} \times \text{Volume drug is in (stock solution)}$$

Worked example

Paracetamol 100mg is prescribed, and you have available paracetamol 250mg/5mL suspension.

The calculation is:

$$\frac{100mg \ (what \ you \ want)}{250mg \ (what \ you \ have \ got)} \times 5mL \ (volume \ drug \ is \ in) = 2mL$$

You would administer 2mL of paracetamol suspension.

Worked example

Paracetamol 100mg is prescribed, and you have available paracetamol 120mg/5mL suspension.

The calculation is:

$$\frac{100mg \ (what \ you \ want)}{120mg \ (what \ you \ have \ got)} \times 5mL \ (volume \ drug \ is \ in) = 4.16mL$$

You would need to administer 4.16mL of paracetamol suspension.

Activity 1.9

Try the following calculations:

1. Paracetamol 60mg   Drug comes as 120mg/5mL.
2. Flucloxacillin 62.5mg   Drug comes as 125mg/5mL.
3. Cefradine 125mg   Drug comes as 250mg/5mL.
4. Phenobarbital 12mg   Drug comes as 15mg/5mL.
5. Prochlorperazine 1.25mg   Drug comes as 5mg/5mL.

continued opposite . . .

continued . . .

6. Morphine 4mg   Drug comes as 10mg/5mL.
7. Phenytoin 75mg   Drug comes as 30mg/5mL.
8. Digoxin 40 micrograms   Drug comes as 50 micrograms/mL (measure with pipette).

Answers are provided at the end of the chapter.

You should practise these calculations until you are comfortable that you can work them out easily. If you are struggling, you should seek further help and advice. Remember to do a mental estimate of what a reasonable answer would be before completing the calculation.

Calculating a dose by body weight

You need to be able to calculate a drug according to body weight in order to check that the prescribed dose and calculation are correct. You must do this before administering any drug, as you are accountable for administering an incorrect dose. You can check the prescription against the recommended dose/kg for that drug in the BNFC.

Worked example

A child weighs 12kg and is prescribed morphine sulphate 200 micrograms/kg.

The calculation would be:

12 x 200 = 2400 micrograms.

Morphine sulphate is available as 10mg/5ml oral solution.

You should have identified in this example that the units involved are different; the dose is in micrograms and the solution in milligrams. To calculate how much to administer we need to convert to the same units.

Worked example

We can convert micrograms to grams by dividing by 1000:

$2400 ÷ 1000 = 2.4g.$

To calculate the volume to administer, apply the formula:

$$\frac{What\ you\ want\ (strength\ required)}{What\ you\ have\ got\ (strength\ available)} \times \begin{array}{c} Volume\ drug\ is\ in \\ (stock\ solution) \end{array}$$

$$\frac{2.4}{10} \times 5 = 1.2$$

Therefore you would administer 1.2mL.

The following activity should familiarise you with calculating doses according to a child's weight.

Activity 1.10

Calculate the dose that should be prescribed in the following cases.

1. Susan weighs 13kg and is prescribed sodium valproate 5mg/kg.
2. James weighs 22kg and is prescribed prednisolone 2mg/kg.
3. Ben weighs 8.2kg and is prescribed phenytoin 1.5mg/kg.

Answers are provided at the end of the chapter.

Expressing strengths in different ways

For some products, the strength of a medicine is not expressed directly in units of weight and volume. The strength may be expressed in a traditional way as the number of parts of the active drug in a given volume. For example, adrenaline injection is generally expressed as 1 in 1000 (1g in 1000mL) or as 1 in 10,000 (1g in 10,000 mL).

It is important for you to understand how to convert 1 in 1000 to mg per mL or micrograms per mL, as you may need to administer a dose in micrograms to a small baby in anaphylactic shock.

Worked example

- 1 in 1000 means that 1g of the active drug is contained in 1000mL of the injection solution.
- 1g in 1000mL = 1000mg in 1000mL.

Divide both by 1000:

- 1000mg in 1000mL = 1mg in 1mL.
- Converting mg to micrograms, 1000 micrograms is in 1mL.

It is usual for the 1 in 1000 strength of adrenaline to be used for children in anaphylactic shock and you will find a table of recommended doses with the volume calculated in the BNFC under 'Allergic emergencies'. Also, see Chapter 6 of this book for management of anaphylaxis.

You may find yourself in a situation where you have to work out the volume, or explain the calculation to others such as parents. The following activity is to check your understanding of this and to provide practice in converting the weights and volumes.

Activity 1.11

Now use the same approach as above to calculate how many micrograms are contained in 1mL of adrenaline 1 in 10 000 solution.

An answer is provided at the end of the chapter.

Now that you are able to convert the solution to more manageable volumes, try the following calculations used in the management of anaphylaxis in children.

Activity 1.12

Calculate the volume of adrenaline 1 in 1000 solution you would administer in order to give the following doses prescribed for anaphylactic shock.

1. 50 micrograms
2. 120 micrograms
3. 250 micrograms
4. 500 micrograms

Answers are provided at the end of the chapter.

You should practise these calculations until you are comfortable that you can work them out easily. You need to feel confident in an emergency situation that you are giving the correct dose.

Always remember to use a suitable syringe for measuring small volumes.

Percentages

In some medicines, the strength of the active ingredient is expressed as a percentage, meaning the number of parts per hundred. For example, glucose 5 per cent (%) solution is an expressive label to describe the fact there are 5 parts of glucose per 100 parts of water. In this case 'per cent' means parts 'per 100'.

Parts per hundred can be expressed in four ways.

For a mixture of two solids, the percentage is expressed as weight in weight (w/w):

- 10% w/w means 10g of an ingredient in 100g of product.

For solids dissolved or suspended in a liquid, the percentage is expressed as weight in volume (w/v):

- 10% w/v means 10g of an ingredient is present in 100mL of solution.

For liquids diluted in another liquid, the percentage is expressed as volume in volume (v/v):

- 10% v/v means 10mL of an ingredient is present in 100mL of product.

For liquids diluted within a solid, the percentage is expressed as volume in weight (v/w):

- 10% v/w means 10mL of an ingredient is present in 100g of product.

The following worked example is to demonstrate how to calculate the amount if the active ingredient is available per mL.

Worked example

- 1% lidocaine (w/v)
- 1% means 1 part of lidocaine in 100 mL of water.
- 1% lidocaine means 1g in 100ml.

We can further divide this down, in order to be able to calculate how much lidocaine is in 1mL, by first converting to mg.

- 1g = 1000mg, so
- 1000mg is in 100mL.

continued opposite . . .

continued . . .

Divide both by 100 to get

- 10mg in 1mL (10mg/mL).

When referring to the BNFC, you will find that next to the product's name and percentage value is the weight per volume value in brackets, for example:

Lidocaine hydrochloride 0.1% (1mg/mL).

Molarity

Another way of expressing the strength of a medicine is by molarity, which uses the theory of basic chemistry. Each atom has an atomic weight, for example sodium (Na) is 23 and chlorine (Cl) is 35.4. When atoms combine together to form molecules, such as sodium and chlorine combining to form sodium chloride (NaCl), the molecular weight is the sum of their combined atomic weights:

Na (23) + Cl (35.4) = NaCl = 58.4.

One **mole** of a drug weighs the same (in grams) as the relative molecular weight for that drug. So, for NaCL, 1 mole weighs 58.4g.

A **molar solution** contains 1 mole per 1 litre. So, in a molar solution of sodium chloride, there is 58.4g NaCl in 1 litre.

The **molarity of a solution** is the number of moles of a substance dissolved in one litre of solution. Thus, a one molar solution of sodium chloride (written as 1M NaCl) has one mole (58.4g) of sodium chloride in one litre of solution.

The strength of pharmaceutical solutions used in electrolyte replacement therapy is normally expressed in mmol/given volume of solution. A mmol is an abbreviation for millimole, which is one-thousandth of a mole.

To calculate the number of millimoles in a solution look at the following worked example.

Worked example

- Sodium chloride 0.9% w/v intravenous solution is commonly administered.
- 0.9g of sodium chloride is in 100mL.

continued overleaf . . .

continued . . .

- $0.9g = 900mg$.
- $900mg$ is in $100mL$ of a solution.

  Intravenous infusions of 0.9% sodium chloride are usually supplied in 1 litre bags

- $9000mg$ is in $1000mL$.

  Therefore, the number of millimoles per litre can be calculated by the molecular weight:

- $\dfrac{9000}{58.4} = 154mmol$ per litre.

Children's nurses will not generally be required to calculate moles or millimoles from first principles, but may have to calculate how much of a given solution to administer where the strength is expressed in mmols/litre. The BNFC provides mmol/litre information next to product information, for example sodium chloride 0.18% (Na+ and Cl– each 30mmol/litre).

Displacement values

Some drugs come in dry powder form and have to be reconstituted with a **diluent** before administration. An example of this is some intravenous antibiotics. The final volume of the solution will be greater than the volume of liquid that was added to the powder. This volume difference is called the displacement value. Displacement values of the dry powder may be significant when reconstituting. For some patients this does not matter because the whole vial is administered, but it is very important in paediatrics and neonatology when you want to give a dose that is less than the total contents of the vial.

Worked example

- Christie has been prescribed $350mg$ of co-amoxiclav injection.
- A $1.2g$ vial of co-amoxiclav has a displacement value of $0.9mL$.

continued opposite . . .

continued . . .

- A 1.2gr vial is normally reconstituted to produce a solution of 1.2gr/20mL.
- You would need to add 19.1mL of water for injection to produce a solution of 1.2gr/20mL.
- 1.2gr is converted to 1200mg/20mL.
- $\dfrac{350}{1200} \times 20 = 5.83mL.$

You can check your answer by estimation; a quarter of the solution would be 300mg in 5mL, so 350mg in 5.83mL is a sensible answer.

You must consult the product guidelines for instructions on how much diluent to add; otherwise the correct dose would not be administered and could lead to a serious error in very small babies. Displacement values vary and depend on the drug, manufacturer and its strength.

Fluid calculations

When nursing adult patients, intravenous fluids are often delivered in number of litres per hour, using standard intravenous administration sets that use gravity to deliver the fluid. The nurse can calculate the number of drops needed per minute to deliver this fluid. As infusion pumps are always recommended to deliver intravenous fluids to children, the formula is only briefly covered in this text, so please refer to the adult book in this series for further information. It is useful for you to know that most standard intravenous administration sets are designed to deliver 1mL in 20 drops of fluid. Therefore, the rate of flow required (number of drops per minute) can be calculated thus:

$$\frac{\text{Volume of fluid (mL)} \times 20}{\text{Duration (min)}} = \text{drops/minute.}$$

Thus, if a child is prescribed 500mL of fluid to run over 8 hours, to calculate the number of drops per minute:

- Convert 8 hours into minutes: $8 \times 60 = 480$.

$$\frac{500 \times 20}{480} = 21 \text{ drops per minute}$$

Correct fluid calculation is an essential skill for all nurses caring for children and they must demonstrate the skills needed to administer medicines safely via various means, including intravenous infusion (ESC 38, NMC, 2010a). Children's nurses need to be able to calculate the hourly rate for intravenous infusions. As with other medicines, you must consider the dosage, weight, method of administration and timing (NMC, 2010b).

Fluids prescribed must be checked, taking into consideration all the fluids the child is receiving, which includes all oral fluids and all intravenous fluids. A number of factors need to be taken into consideration when deciding a child's **maintenance fluids**, including age and weight, so you should check your local guidelines for intravenous fluid administration.

Table 1.4 is an example of baseline fluid requirements for children of different ages. Conditions of increased fluid loss (burns and pyrexia) and reduced fluid loss (renal failure, hypothermia, high ambient humidity) need to be taken into consideration when estimating fluid needs.

Body weight	24-hour fluid requirement
Under 10kg	100mL/kg
Over 20kg	100mL/kg for the first 10kg
	+ 50mL/kg for each kg between 10 and 20kg
	+ 20mL/kg for each 1kg body weight over 20kg
	(max. 2 litres in females, 2.5 litres in males)

Table 1.4: Fluid requirements for children over 1 month (BMA et al., 2010)

Worked example

A baby weighs 6kg and the maintenance fluid required is 100ml/kg/24 hours. What is the hourly rate for the intravenous infusion?

- Requirement for 24 hours is 6 x 100mL = 600mL.
- Requirement per hour is 600 ÷ 24 = 25mL per hour.

Sometimes, because of certain clinical conditions, fluid requirements need to be reduced by a percentage of their usual daily requirements.

Worked example

The maintenance fluid requirement is 500mL per 24 hours. A baby is prescribed 75% of the maintenance fluid, so what will be the hourly rate?

continued opposite . . .

continued . . .

- 75% of 500mL = 375mL ÷ 24 = 15.63ml/hr (to 2 decimal places).

The following activity is to help you to improve your skill in calculating different types of fluid prescriptions, and to practise calculating intravenous fluid rates and feed volumes to meet total maintenance requirements.

Activity 1.13

1. A child is prescribed 500mL of intravenous fluid to be given over 8 hours. What is the hourly rate?

2. A baby weighs 4.6kg and the maintenance fluid requirements are 100mL/kg/24 hours. You need to give 3-hourly feeds using 75 per cent of the maintenance requirements. The other 25 per cent of maintenance requirements will be given intravenously. How much oral feed will you be giving 3-hourly and what will be the intravenous infusion rate?

3. A 3kg baby has an intravenous infusion running at 5mL per hour. The maintenance requirements for this baby are 100mL per kilogram per 24 hours. The baby is also receiving a bolus injection of 5.5mL of drugs every 6 hours. What volume of feed should be given hourly?

Answers are provided at the end of the chapter.

Since your calculations can have important consequences for your patients, double-check your answers by working your calculation backwards to see if you get the same quantities. You will find in some areas of practice that you will be required to make many such calculations on a daily basis. Check your answer with a colleague and, if you are unable to agree, ask a third person such as a doctor or pharmacist.

Checking the correct dose

Before you administer a drug to a child you must be sure that the prescribed dose is correct. You must have considered the dosage, weight where appropriate, method of administration, route and timing (Standard 8, NMC, 2010b). You cannot assume that the prescriber is correct. Always be aware that someone could have made a mistake when they wrote the child's weight on the drug chart. Assess the weight on the chart; does it make sense for the age of the child? If you are unsure, check using a growth chart. Next, check in the BNFC the recommended dose r kilogram for the prescribed drug. If there is a discrepancy, do not give the drug but check the prescriber.

The next activity is to familiarise you with the routine of checking drug dosages before administration.

Activity 1.14

Check these prescribed doses using the BNFC, which you can access online at **www.bnfc.org/bnfc**. Would you administer them?

1. Fiona is 13 years old and has fallen off her pony and fractured her wrist. She weighs 40kg and is prescribed paracetamol 500mg every 4–6 hours.
2. Josh is 9 years old and has attended due to an acute asthmatic attack. He weighs 3kg and has been prescribed oral prednisolone 6mg once daily for 5 days.
3. Sam is 3 days old and has been diagnosed with a urinary tract infection for which he has been prescribed amoxicillin. His weight is 3.2kg and he is prescribed amoxicillin 96mg 3 times daily.
4. Marnell is 15 years old and weighs 58kg. She has acute tonsillitis for which she has been prescribed phenoxymethylpenicillin (penicillin v) 250mg 4 times daily.

Answers are provided at the end of the chapter.

Chapter summary

You should now be aware of how drugs are calculated and prescribed according to a child's weight or body surface area. You should feel comfortable with the metric system and SI units and how to convert one unit of measurement into another. The chapter has enabled you to estimate a child's weight in an emergency and calculate children's drug doses. When calculating drug doses you will now form the safe habit of estimating the dose in order to check it is correct. You should also now feel confident in calculating the fluid requirements and intravenous infusion rates for children.

Activities: brief outline answers

Activity 1.1 (pages 9–10)

1. 250 micrograms = 0.25 milligrams
2. 1345 milligrams = 1,345,000 micrograms
3. 3000 nanograms = 3 micrograms
4. 1.34 kilograms = 1340 grams
5. 145g = 0.145 kilograms
6. 0.07g = 70 milligrams
7. 0.45 micrograms = 450 nanograms
8. 500 milligrams = 0.5 grams

Activity 1.2 (page 10)

1. 500mL = 0.5L
2. 1.2L = 1200ml
3. 30mL = 30,000 microlitres
4. 6000 microlitres = 6mL

Activity 1.3 (page 12)

The answer is 1mL of Nystan suspension, which is supplied with a pipette for measurement.

Activity 1.4 (page 14)

1. Weight = $2 \times (2 + 4) = 2 \times 6 = 12$kg
2. Weight = $2 \times (6 + 4) = 2 \times 10 = 20$kg
3. Weight = $2 \times (10 + 4) = 2 \times 14 = 28$kg
4. Weight = $2 \times (5 + 4) = 2 \times 9 = 18$kg

Activity 1.5 (page 16)

1. You need to convert the ounces into a decimal; 12 ounces is 12/16 of a pound = 0.75, so 7.75lb ÷ 2.2 = 3.52kg.
2. 3 stone into lb is $3 \times 14 = 42$lb; then 42 ÷ 2.2 = 19.09kg.
3. 1 stone 8lb = 14 + 8 = 22lb; then 22 ÷ 2.2 = 10kg.
4. 3.6kg $\times 2.2 = 7.92$lb. Convert 0.92lb to ounces: 0.92×16oz = 14.72oz. Answer is 7lb 15oz (to the nearest ounce).
5. 24.5kg $\times 2.2 = 53.9$lb. Convert 0.9lb to ounces: 0.9×16oz = 14.4oz. Answer is 53lb 14oz (to the nearest ounce).

Activity 1.6 (page 19)

Have you ever heard or said any of the following?

- 'I can't understand that.'
- 'Are you sure?'
- 'Let's just get a move on, we haven't got time.'
- 'I'm in charge here; I know what I'm doing.'

Have you ever had the feeling that something is just not right?

If so, you must act to prevent a potential medication error.

Challenge opinion, ask for more information and alert others.

You should never feel pressured to trust a more experienced or senior colleague when you disagree. You should always ask for a third person, perhaps a doctor or pharmacist, when there is a calculation discrepancy. Do not be pressured by time restraints; prioritise getting it right, and allow the time.

The evidence for single-nurse administration being more effective and efficient as opposed to double-checking is inconclusive. Be guided by local policy.

Activity 1.7 (page 22)

1. $\dfrac{240}{120} = 2$ tablets

2. $\dfrac{300}{100} = 3$ tablets

3. $\dfrac{40}{5} = 8$ tablets

4. $\dfrac{4}{2} = 2$ tablets

Activity 1.8 (page 23)

1. First convert to the same units, 0.25mg = 250 micrograms, so you would need to give 1 tablet.
2. Again, convert 1g to mg =1000mg. Now calculate how many capsules either by using the formula, or mental arithmetic:

$$\dfrac{1000}{250} = 4 \text{ capsules.}$$

3. Convert 0.5g to mg = 500mg; 2 × 250mg tablets would equal 500mg.

Activity 1.9 (page 24)

1. $\dfrac{60}{120} \times 5 = 2.5\text{mL}$

2. $\dfrac{62.5}{125} \times 5 = 2.5\text{mL}$

3. $\dfrac{125}{250} \times 5 = 2.5\text{mL}$

4. $\dfrac{12}{15} \times 5 = 4\text{mL}$

5. $\dfrac{1.25}{5} \times 5 = 1.25\text{mL}$

6. $\dfrac{4}{10} \times 5 = 2\text{mL}$

7. $\dfrac{75}{30} \times 5 = 12.5\text{mL}$

8. $\dfrac{40}{50} \times 1 = 0.8\text{mL}$

Did you check these answers against your mental estimate? How close were your answers?

Activity 1.10 (page 26)

1. Susan 13 × 5 = 65mg
2. James 22 × 2 = 44mg
3. Ben 8.2 × 1.5 = 12.3mg

Activity 1.11 (page 27)

- 1 in 10,000 means that 1g of the active drug is contained in 10,000mL of the injection solution.
- 1g in 10,000mL = 1000mg in 10,000mL.

If you then divide both by 1000:

- 1000mg in 10,000mL = 1mg in 10mL.

Convert to micrograms:

- 1000 micrograms in 10mL.
- 100 micrograms in 1mL.

Activity 1.12 (page 27)

First we need to establish that 1 in 1000 solution contains 1000 microgram in 1ml.

1. $\dfrac{50}{1000} \times 1 = 0.05\text{mL}$

2. $\dfrac{120}{1000} \times 1 = 0.12\text{mL}$

3. $\dfrac{250}{1000} \times 1 = 0.25\text{mL}$

4. $\dfrac{500}{1000} \times 1 = 0.5\text{mL}$

Activity 1.13 (page 33)

1. $500 \div 8 = 62.5\text{mL}$ per hour.
2. Total fluid requirement per 24 hours is $4.6 \times 100 = 460\text{mL}$.
   Intravenous requirement $25\% \times 460 = 115\text{mL}$.
   Hourly intravenous rate $115 \div 24 = 4.8\text{mL}$ per hour (to nearest decimal place).
   Oral requirement $75\% \times 460 = 345\text{mL}$ per 24 hours.
   345mL $\div$ 8 feeds in 24 hours = 43mL every 3 hours (to nearest decimal place).
3. Total 24 hr requirement $3 \times 100 = 300\text{mL}$ per 24 hours.
   Total IV volume per 24 hours is $5 \times 24 = 120\text{mL}$ plus bolus ($4 \times 5.5 = 22$) = 142mL.
   Fluid deficit to be given orally is $300 - 142 = 158\text{mL}$.
   Hourly feeds $158 \div 24 = 6.58\text{mL}$ rounded to 6.6mL.

Activity 1.14 (page 34)

1. Fiona. This would seem to be a reasonable weight and dose for a 13-year-old child; 40kg is on the twenty-fifth centile for a 13-year-old girl, so in practice you would be able to visualise that she is below average for her age. The dose of paracetamol for a child of 12–18 years is 500mg every 4–6 hours.
2. Josh. This dose of prednisolone is much too small for a child with acute asthma aged 9 years. Note his weight – 3kg is below average for a newborn baby. Josh's weight was 30kg, but the nurse had omitted the zero when transcribing to the drug chart. A child aged 2–18 years with acute asthma should be prescribed prednisolone oral 1–2mg/kg (max. 40mg) once daily 3–5 days. The correct dose would be between 30mg and 40mg prednisolone oral once daily 3–5 days.
3. Sam. You should stop and question this prescription. Neonates are the group most vulnerable to drug errors, so you should be extra vigilant. A weight of 3.2kg is reasonable for a 3-day-old male infant. The oral dose for amoxicillin for a nenoate under 7 days is 30mg/kg (so 96mg would be the correct calculation); however, maximum dose is 62.5mg TWICE daily. The drug has been prescribed 3 times daily, which is an error. Neonates clear drugs from their system much slower due to immature kidneys, so require less frequent dosing. The dose can be doubled in severe infection, but this still wouldn't be correct. You cannot assume it was the intention of the prescriber to double the dose; you should not administer the drug and should check with the prescriber.
4. Marnell. The correct dose for a child aged 12–18 years of phenoxymethylpenicillin (penicillin v) is 500mg 4 times daily; increased in severe infection up to 1g 4 times daily. A weight of 58kg is reasonable for a 15-year-old female.

Further reading

Hutton, M and Gardner, H (2005) Calculation skills. *Paediatric Nursing*, 17(2) (March).

This is a guide for all nurses working with neonates, children and young people to support their learning and revision of calculation skills. It provides guidance and practical exercises for commonly encountered problems and is available online at **www.cardiff.ac.uk/mathssupport/learningresources/ mathsforhealth/pncalculationskills.pdf**.

Downie, G, Mackenzie, J and Williams, A (2006) *Calculating Drug Doses Safely: A handbook for nurses and midwives*. Edinburgh: Churchill Livingstone.

This book covers revision of arithmetic in a stepwise approach for you to proceed at your own pace. It contains actual medicine labels in order for you to relate theory to practice, with some more advanced material to suit a range of abilities.

Useful websites

www.bnfc.org/bnfc

This website provides access to the complete text of the *British National Formulary for Children*. Registration is free for NHS personnel. Resources include online calculators for imperial–metric conversion and body mass index.

Chapter 2
Legal and ethical issues in children's medicines management

continued . . . ••

6. Fully understands the different types of prescribing including supplementary prescribing, community practitioner nurse prescribing and independent nurse prescribing.

42. People can trust the newly registered graduate nurse to demonstrate understanding and knowledge to supply and administer via a patient group direction.

By the second progression point:

1. Demonstrates knowledge of what a patient group direction is and who can use them.

By entry to the register:

2. **Through simulation and course work** demonstrates knowledge and application of the principles required for safe and effective supply and administration via a patient group direction including an understanding of role and accountability.

3. **Through simulation and course work** demonstrates how to supply and administer via a patient group direction.

Chapter aims

By the end of this chapter, you should be able to:

*   understand the law relating to medicines management and the nurse's accountability;
*   understand the ethical issues relating to medicines and to children and consent;
*   demonstrate knowledge of what a patient group direction (PGD) is and who can use them.

Case studies

In May 1993, it was widely reported that a nurse called Beverley Allitt had been convicted for the murder of four children, attempting to murder another three and causing grievous bodily harm with intent to a further six on the children's ward of Grantham and Kesteven Hospital in Lincolnshire. Allitt murdered the four children by injecting them with high doses of insulin. There was also evidence that some children had been injected with potassium and lignocaine. She was diagnosed with a condition called 'fabricated illness by proxy' and given 13 life sentences. An independent inquiry was held into the deaths and injuries by Sir Cecil Clothier in 1994 (resulting in the Clothier Report), which made 12 recommendations, including stricter criteria for selection and progress in nurse training and clinical supervision for qualified nurses.

In January 2000, Dr Harold Shipman was convicted of murdering 15 of his patients while working as a GP in Manchester, and it is believed he may have murdered many more by administering lethal injections of controlled drugs. The Shipman Inquiry investigated how current systems could be changed to safeguard patients.

continued opposite . . .

continued . . .

> *The law in relation to medicines has been shaped by such incidents and is designed to protect the public and practitioners from the clear potential dangers.*
>
> *The Fourth Report of the House of Commons Select Committee on Health,* The Regulation of Controlled Drugs in the Community *(2004), resulting from the Shipman Inquiry, influenced the systems of management and regulation of controlled drugs, together with the conduct for those who operate those systems.*

Introduction

The Nursing and Midwifery Council *Standards for Medicines Management* (2010b) are explicit in the expectations of registered nurses, and *The Code* (NMC, 2008) applies as much to medicines management as to any other aspect of nursing care. It is expected that registered nurses are accountable for their practice and always act lawfully both in professional practice and personal life (NMC, 2008). In order to act within the law, it is essential that you have an awareness and knowledge of the law of the country within which you practise.

This chapter will outline the law as it relates to medicines management. However, it cannot cover everything you will need to know. The law changes frequently, particularly in relation to medicines and non-medical prescribing. It is important that you keep yourself up to date with current practice. You must also make yourself aware of any local policies within your area of work relating to procedures for the administration and storage of medicines. These policies are derived from statutory sources and guidance issued by the Department of Health.

This chapter will also discuss the complexity of consent, and some of the ethical issues associated with medicines and children.

The law and medicines administration

The manufacture, storage, distribution, labelling and sale of drugs are controlled by legislation that aims to protect patients from harm arising from inappropriate use. The legislation also aims to provide nurses and other healthcare professionals, such as doctors, pharmacists and dentists, with a comprehensive framework for their clinical practice.

The Medicines Act 1968

The Medicines Act 1968 was the first comprehensive legislation in the UK that, along with secondary legislation, controls the regulation, manufacture, distribution and importation of all medicines for both human and animal use. Also established in 1968 was the Medicines Commission, which advises government health ministers on the implementation of the Medicines Act.

In 2005 the Medicines and Healthcare products Regulatory Agency (MHRA) undertook a public consultation to amend the advisory structure of the Medicines Act 1968. A new structure was agreed, amalgamating the responsibilities of the Medicines Commission and the Committee on Safety of Medicines to become the Commission on Human Medicines. The duties of the Commission are set out in Section 3 of the Medicines Act 1968 (as amended by the Medicines Advisory Bodies Regulations 2005). These duties include the following.

- To advise ministers on matters relating to human medicines (except those that fall under the remit of the Advisory Board on the Registration of Homeopathic Products (ABRH) and Herbal Medicines Advisory Committee (HMAC).
- To advise the licensing authority, including giving advice on safety, quality and effectiveness of human medicines.
- To promote the collection and investigation of information in relation to adverse reactions to medicines (except for those products that fall within the remit of the ABRH or HMAC) for the purpose of enabling advice to be given.

The Medicines Act 1968 identified the following three categories of drug products.

1. **General sales list (GSL) medicines**
   This refers to the category of licensed medicines that do not require a prescription and that may be sold to the public without the supervision of a pharmacist under certain conditions. These medicines can be sold in such places as supermarkets and shops, provided that the premises can be locked and that the medicines are prepacked elsewhere and not previously opened.

2. **Pharmacy (P) medicines**
   Pharmacy medicines do not require a prescription but can only be sold or supplied to the public at a registered pharmacy by, or under the supervision of, a pharmacist.

3. **Prescription-only medicines (POMs)**
   POMs are those products that may only be sold or supplied in accordance with a **prescription** given by an appropriate practitioner. An appropriate practitioner in the UK may be a doctor, dentist or non-medical prescriber, such as a supplementary prescriber or pharmacist or nurse independent prescriber. A person may not administer a POM, except to themselves, unless they are an appropriate practitioner or acting in accordance with the directions of the appropriate practitioner.

The following section will now look at medicines within the different categories and the law in relation to drugs.

There are exceptions to this ruling to allow for emergencies made under the Prescription Only Medicines (Human Use) Order 1997 (and subsequent Amendment Orders 2001 and 2003). According to this Order, some medicines for use by **parenteral** administration are exempt from this restriction when given to save life in an emergency. This means there are specific prescription-only medicines that can be administered without a prescription in certain emergency situations such as anaphylactic shock and hypoglycaemic episodes. They include:

- glucagon injection;
- adrenaline injection 1 in 1000;
- atropine sulphate injection;

- promethazine hydrochloride injection;
- hydrocortisone injection;
- chlorpheniramine injection;
- snake venom antiserum.

Some midwives may also administer certain POMs under exemption, such as oxytocin and pethidine, in the course of their professional practice. Paramedics may administer certain POMs, such as naloxene and diazemuls, if they hold a certificate of proficiency in paramedical skills issued under approval of the Secretary of State.

The way medicines fall into one of these categories of medicines can be very complicated. The category may differ according to the route of administration, or the condition for which it is being used. You would not be expected to learn the category of every medicine available, but you should be knowledgeable of those medicines that are commonly used within your field of practice.

The following activity will help you to identify the category of common medicines used in children and appreciate the importance of checking each individual medicine according to the route and use.

Activity 2.1	*Evidence-based practice and research*

Using the *British National Formulary for Children* (BNFC), search for the following commonly used drugs and identify if they are a prescription-only medicine by looking for the following symbol: PoM :

- amoxicillin;
- chlorphenamine maleate;
- hydrocortisone cream.

Outline answers are provided at the end of the chapter.

Homeopathic medicines

Homeopathic medicines in the UK are currently covered by either Product Licences of Rights (PLRs), issued to all medicines on the market when the Medicines Act 1968 was introduced, or by certificates of registration under the Simplified Registration Scheme. The National Rules Scheme for homeopathic medicines was introduced in 2006 in order to build on the existing regulatory framework. The National Rules Scheme places particular emphasis on indications and appropriate labelling literature. All homeopathic medicines fall within the scope of the Yellow Card Scheme, allowing patients and healthcare professionals to report suspected side effects of homeopathic medicines to the MHRA (see **www.yellowcard.gov.uk**).

Herbal medicines

Not all herbal medicines are regulated by the MHRA and therefore do not necessarily meet assured safety standards. Those that are regulated have Product Licence (PL) numbers on their labels. The MHRA launched a registration scheme for herbal medicines in 2005 called the Traditional Herbal Registration (THR) scheme. Under this scheme, herbal medicines have to be produced to meet specific standards of safety and quality and have THR numbers on their labels.

A herbal remedy without a PL or THR number on its label is unlicensed and has *not* been assessed by the MHRA, and therefore nothing is known about its safety, quality or any potential side effects.

Companies with existing unlicensed herbal medicines on the market have to register them with the MHRA under the THR scheme by 2011. It is still permitted in the UK under the Medicines Act 1968 for herbal remedies that have been manufactured on a person's premises to be supplied to patients following individual consultation. The process of producing the herbal remedy must only consist of the drying, crushing or chopping up of plants. The remedy must be sold without any written recommendation for its use and must not be given a name other than the plant and process (e.g. powdered rose hips).

The Misuse of Drugs Act 1971

The Misuse of Drugs Act 1971 controls the export, import, production, supply and possession of drugs that are dangerous or otherwise harmful. The Act renders unlawful all activities in the drugs controlled under the Act, except those provided for under the regulations made under the Act. The drugs subject to the control of the Act are termed 'controlled drugs' (CDs) and are listed in Schedule 2 of the Act. These drugs are further divided into classes A, B and C, on the basis of decreasing harmfulness. The classes are for the purpose of establishing maximum penalties that can be imposed for offences under the Act and are not directly relevant to patient care. Here are some examples of CDs in each class:

- Class A: diamorphine, cocaine, LSD, methadone;
- Class B: codeine, amphetamines;
- Class C: diazepam, anabolic steroids.

In practice, you may at times use diamorphine and codeine for acute or chronic pain. Methadone is sometimes the drug of dependence in neonatal abstinence syndrome and can be used in babies of mothers who have been taking it during pregnancy. Amphetamines are stimulants (street name 'speed') that cause wakefulness and excessive activity. They are sometimes used for the management of attention deficit hyperactivity disorder (ADHD) (dexamphetamine sulphate). The prescribing of amphetamines has now reduced because of illicit use. Diazepam is rarely used in children and only to relieve acute anxiety and insomnia caused by fear (such as before surgery).

The Misuse of Drugs Regulations 2001

The use of controlled drugs in medicine is permitted under the Misuse of Drugs Regulations 2001, the current version made under the Misuse of Drugs Act 1971 (2001 Regulations). The Regulations are periodically updated and amended and those currently in force are available at the Office for Public Sector Information (OPSI) website (see 'Useful websites' at the end of the chapter). A list of drugs controlled under the misuse of drugs legislation, including their classification under both the Misuse of Drugs Act 1971 and the Misuse of Drugs Regulations 2001, is available on the Home Office website, again given at the end of the chapter.

The Misuse of Drugs Regulations 2001 divide CDs into five schedules that dictate the degree to which their use is regulated. The schedule within which the CD is placed is a balance of the benefit of the drug's therapeutic effect against the harm it causes when misused. Schedule 1 CDs are subject to the highest level of control, whereas Schedule 5 CDs are subject to a much lower level of control.

Schedule 1 (CD Licence)

Schedule 1 drugs have no recognised medicinal use and include such drugs as hallucinogenics. Practitioners, including doctors, dentists and veterinary practitioners, may not lawfully possess Schedule 1 drugs unless they have a special licence to do so from the Home Office, for specific purposes such as research.

Examples of Schedule 1 drugs are:

- cannabis
- cannabis resin
- coca leaf
- lysergide
- N-alkyl derivatives of lysergamide.

Schedule 2 (CD POM)

This includes drugs such as major stimulants and opioids. A licence is required to import or export Schedule 2 drugs.

Examples of Schedule 2 drugs are:

- methadone
- morphine
- cocaine
- diamorphine.

Schedule 2 CDs may be administered to a patient by any person authorised to prescribe them, or by any person acting in accordance with the directions of an appropriate person authorised to prescribe CDs. This includes nurse independent prescribers, who are currently permitted to prescribe, administer and direct others to administer certain CDs for specific conditions and routes of administration.

Schedule 3 (CD No Register)

This includes drugs such as minor stimulants that are thought to be less likely to be misused, or less harmful when misused than drugs in Schedule 2. Schedule 3 drugs are exempt from safe custody requirements; however, temazepam, flunitrazepam, buprenorphine and diethylpropion are exceptions that must be stored in a CD cupboard in a secure environment.

Examples of Schedule 3 drugs are:

- temazepam
- buprenorphine
- phentermine.

Schedule 4 (CD benzodiazepines and anabolic steroids)

This schedule has two parts. In part I are benzodiazepines and other substances, while part II contains anabolic steroids and androgenic steroids, as well as other substances. It is an offence to possess a drug from Schedule 4, part I, without an appropriate prescription. There is no restriction on the possession of a part II CD anabolic steroid drug when it is part of a medicinal product.

Examples of Schedule 4, part I, drugs are:

- clonazepam
- tetrazepam
- nitrazepam.

Examples of Schedule 4, part II, drugs are:

- mesterolone
- testosterone
- nandrolone.

Schedule 5 (CD Invoice)

These are preparations that contain low strengths of certain CDs, such as codeine and morphine, but are exempt from full control as the risk of misuse is reduced. There are no restrictions on their possession, import, export or administration or destruction, and safe custody regulations do not apply. However, invoices for these preparations must be kept for at least two years.

Examples of Schedule 5 drugs are:

- preparations containing not more than 0.1 per cent cocaine;
- preparations containing not more than 0.2 per cent morphine.

The following activity will help you to identify the schedules that different drugs fall into.

Activity 2.2   *Evidence-based practice and research*

Follow the link **www.legislation.gov.uksi/2001/3998/contents/made** to the Misuse of Drugs Regulations 2001 in order to identify the schedules of the following drugs:

- phentermine
- lorazepam
- pethidine
- fentanyl.

Outline answers are provided at the end of the chapter.

Safe custody

The senior registered nurse or acting senior registered nurse in charge of a hospital ward or department has responsibility for the possession, safe custody and issue of controlled drugs under The Misuse of Drugs (Safe Custody) Regulations 1973 and subsequent Misuse of Drugs Regulations 2001 and Misuse of Drugs (Safe Custody) (amendment) Regulations 2007.

The CDs must be stored in a locked container, such as a CD cabinet or safe, which can only be opened by the person in lawful possession of the CD, that is, the senior registered nurse or acting senior registered nurse. For practical reasons, to ensure that CDs are always readily available to patients, the senior registered nurse or acting senior registered nurse in charge may delegate the control of access to another registered nurse or sometimes medical practitioner (such as an anaesthetist or paediatrician). This access must be strictly controlled in practice and set out in locally agreed guidelines. The responsibility for all CDs remains with the senior registered nurse on duty, even if the nurse allows access by others. The Misuse of Drugs (Safe Custody) (amendment) Regulations 2007 allows operating department practitioners to order, possess and supply CDs.

The safe storage of Schedule 2 drugs in the community

If drugs are stored on GP surgery premises:

- CDs should be stored in a safe cabinet under lock and key;
- the locked cabinet should preferably be steel, fixed to a wall or the floor, ideally within another cupboard to avoid easy detection by intruders, and the room containing the safe cabinet should be lockable;
- walls to the room should be of suitable thickness using suitable material;
- stock should be kept to a minimum;
- nothing should indicate on the outside of the container that controlled drugs are kept inside;
- a locked container is necessary for drugs in transit.

The following scenario highlights the importance of ensuring the safe storage of medicine is closely adhered to when children are about.

Case study

An 11-month-old girl was admitted to an accident and emergency department unwell with symptoms of lethargy. After numerous investigations, including urine toxicology testing, she was diagnosed with methadone intoxication. The grandfather had been babysitting the infant prior to the admission. The grandfather had been prescribed methadone for morphine addiction and he was carrying a 5mg methadone tablet in his pocket. The infant was treated successfully and recovered (Glatstein et al., 2009).

Small children are inquisitive and will often place substances in their mouths. Just one small tablet mislaid can be a real danger to them and potentially fatal.

Healthcare premises such as a hospital wards or a health centre may be more dangerous to children than their own homes. There are many hazards to children in such environments, such as equipment and medicines. They are busy places and supervision of children is not always easy, especially if the areas are overcrowded or short-staffed. All children's nurses should view child safety as a priority and ensure that children are as safe as reasonably possible when on healthcare premises. You should set a good example to parents with your approach to the storage and handling of medicines. You should ensure that parents are given good medicines safety advice when discharged home. Medicines should be kept in a locked cabinet in the home and out of the reach of young children.

Record keeping requirements in respect of drugs in Schedules 2 and 3

A record must be kept in the controlled drugs record book of all Schedule 2 and 3 drugs by any person authorised to supply them. Each CD must have its name specified at the top of the page and its own separate page within the record book. The number of tablets or ampoules for each CD is counted and specified at the top of the page. The date, time, signature of the person who administered the drug, plus the signature of a witness, are recorded with the name of the patient after each administration of the drug. The number of tablets or ampoules is checked against the record book before each administration, and the number remaining after administration is recorded, as a running balance. All entries must be made in ink, and no deletions, obliterations or cancellations can be made. There will be local policies and guidelines as to the frequent checking of these record books against the stock balance of drugs. The purpose is to prevent the misuse of controlled drugs by those who have access to them. This means that, as a registered children's nurse, you should be familiar with the policy concerning schedule 2 drugs such as morphine and schedule 3 drugs such as temazepam within your practice setting. If you are responsible for the storage or administration of CDs, you must have an understanding of your responsibility under the law (NMC, 2004).

Prescriptions

The prescription is an authorised health professional's written instruction for the use of a medicine and must meet the existing legal requirements. A prescription can now be written by a qualified medical, nurse, pharmacist or allied health professional prescriber.

For a prescription to be valid it has to meet the following requirements.

- It is written in ink and indelible (carbon copies of NHS prescriptions are permissible as long as they are signed in ink).
- It is signed and dated by the person issuing it (computer-generated facsimile signatures do not meet legal requirements).
- The dose is specified with the form of the preparation (e.g. liquid, tablet, suppository).
- The full name and address of the patient are given, except for patients in hospital or nursing home situations.
- The age and date of birth of the child are stated.

It is a legal requirement in the case of a prescription-only medicine to state the age of children under 12 years. If any of the above information is missing or invalid, the prescription should be referred back to the prescriber.

Hospital prescription charts

Hospital prescription charts must include the following information:

- the child's full name and hospital number;
- the child's age and date of birth;
- the child's weight in kilograms;
- the hospital and ward.

The following six items must be present as part of the actual prescription before the medication can be given:

- date;
- medicine (written in full);
- dose;
- frequency or time for administration;
- route;
- prescriber's signature in full for each medicine prescribed.

If any of the above information is missing or unclear, do not administer the drug; refer it back to the prescriber to amend the prescription.

Non-medical prescribing

The Medicines Act 1968 only allowed doctors, dentists and veterinary surgeons to prescribe medicines. The Cumberlege Report (DHSS, 1986), on the future of community nursing, made a recommendation that community nurses be allowed to prescribe from a limited list. These recommendations came from a desire to make greater use of the skills and experience of those nurses working in primary and secondary care to make clinical decisions to ensure patients were given timely access to medications and dressings. An 'Advisory Group on Nurse Prescribing' was established, chaired by Dr June Crown, and two Crown Reports followed. Their recommendations are important for community nurses so they are described here in some detail.

Crown Report 1989

The first Crown Report (DH, 1989) recommended that community nurses and health visitors who had completed the necessary training be allowed to prescribe from a limited list. Nurses were also allowed to supply medicines within 'group protocols'. A group protocol was a specific written instruction drawn up locally by doctors and pharmacists to supply or administer a named medicine by other health professionals in a given situation. Examples of this would be group protocols for the nurse-led immunisation of children, or for the adjustment of doses for asthma management. A legal question arose with group protocols as to whether nurses were acting within the law if administering unlicensed and off-label medicines, which is a particular problem within neonates and children. The report recommended that *the law should be clarified to ensure that health professionals who supply or administer medicines under approved group protocols are acting within the law.*

Crown Report 1999

The second Crown Report, *Review of the Prescribing, Supply and Administration of Medicines* (DH, 1999), dealt mainly with the question of professionals other than doctors and dentists initiating and prescribing drugs outside the narrow use of group protocols. The government supported nurse prescribing and announced the intention to train 20,000 health visitors and nurses over two years to make nurse prescribing a reality. The aim was to benefit patient care and enhance patient safety. Because of concerns about the training of nurses and other healthcare professionals in relation to taking a history and physical examination to arrive at a diagnosis, it recommended that two types of prescriber should be recognised.

- Independent prescribing: full responsibility is taken for prescribing a medicine for a patient and for the appropriateness of that prescription. An independent prescriber is accountable and responsible for the assessment of patients with both diagnosed and undiagnosed conditions and for the clinical decision making for the management of those conditions.

For example, an independent nurse prescriber in the community might assess a baby with a sore mouth, diagnose oral thrush and then prescribe nystatin oral suspension.

- Supplementary prescribing (previously known as dependent prescribing): healthcare professionals are authorised to prescribe specified medicines for patients whose condition has been diagnosed by an independent prescriber within an agreed clinical management plan. The supplementary prescriber may issue repeat prescriptions or adjust the dose of medicines according to the management plan and patient needs.

For example, a GP is the independent prescriber and has agreed a clinical management plan with a young person who has chronic asthma, and a practice nurse who is a supplementary prescriber. The practice nurse is able to issue the young person with repeat prescriptions when she performs their asthma review. She is also able to issue prescriptions to 'step up' and 'step down' the treatment according to the young person's clinical needs.

Scenario

Carole is a paediatric community nurse and had been qualified for three years when she decided to train as a supplementary nurse prescriber. This meant that she was able to have agreed clinical management plans with the GPs and paediatricians for some of the children and young people with chronic conditions that she was visiting at home. Carole was able to prescribe antibiotics, corticosteroids and bronchodilators for the children/young people with chronic respiratory conditions when needed, within the guidelines of the clinical management plans. It improved the children's access to medicines, made Carole's job easier and increased her job satisfaction as she felt her skills were being better used. The GP and paediatrician were very happy with this arrangement as they felt the children were receiving the medicines they needed promptly.

continued opposite . . .

continued . . .

Two years later Carole applied to become, and was successfully appointed as, a Paediatric Respiratory Nurse Specialist. In order to fulfil this new role, Carole trained as an independent nurse prescriber. This meant that Carole was able to assess, diagnose and prescribe for those children/young people within her care without the need for a clinical management plan.

Unlicensed medicines

Another recommendation of the Crown Report 1999 was that these newly authorised prescribers would not normally be able to prescribe unlicensed medicines, or medicines outside their licence indication. Pharmaceutical companies do not usually test their medicines on children and therefore cannot apply to license their medicines for use in the treatment of children. It is common practice in paediatrics to prescribe unlicensed medicines and medicines outside the licence to children. A drug company needs a licence to market and promote a drug, but a doctor can prescribe a drug that is not licensed. It is also not illegal for a doctor to prescribe the drug for a different indication of the licence or a different age group. This is called 'off-label' prescribing (see section on 'Off-label medication' below).

As far as is reasonably possible, medicines should be prescribed in accordance with the terms and conditions of their licence. However, there are many instances where children require medicines that are not specifically licensed for paediatric use.

Following review of the legislation on 21 December 2009, qualified nurse and pharmacist independent prescribers are able to prescribe unlicensed medicines on the same basis as doctors and dentists. Nurse independent prescribers are able to prescribe off-label or off-licence medicines where it is best practice to do so, as long as they take full clinical responsibility.

Supplementary prescribing of unlicensed medicine

A nurse, midwife, pharmacist or allied health professional may prescribe unlicensed medication to a child as part of a clinical management plan so long as the following provisions are made.

- The doctor or dentist and the supplementary prescriber have agreed the plan with the child and family in a voluntary relationship.
- An alternative medication would not meet the child's needs.
- There is a sufficient evidence base and/or experience to demonstrate the medication's safety and **efficacy** for that particular child.
- The doctor or dentist is prepared to take the responsibility for prescribing the unlicensed medicine and has agreed the child's clinical management plan to that effect.
- The child and family agree to the prescription in the knowledge that the drug is unlicensed and understand the implications of this.
- The medication and the reasons for choosing the medication are documented in the clinical management plan.
- The doctor or dentist and supplementary prescriber jointly oversee the child's care and monitor and provide any necessary follow-up treatment.

The *British National Formulary for Children* provides advice on the use of unlicensed medicines and the use of licensed medicines for unlicensed use (off-label use). Careful consideration needs to be given to all the options available to manage a given condition, against the available evidence and experience of the unlicensed intervention.

Scenarios

Thomas, who is 4 years old, has been having partial seizures that have not been controlled after trying a number of anti-epileptic medicines. The paediatrician has decided to try gabapentin as an adjunctive treatment to try and control the seizures. Gabapentin is not licensed for use in children under 6 years, but in this case the paediatrician feels that there is no suitable alternative. The paediatrician is using the best evidence available to guide him in prescribing this unlicensed medicine and feels he is able to justify this action.

Evie is a community children's nurse and a qualified independent nurse prescriber. Three-week-old Ruby attends the baby clinic with her mother Lizzie, who is concerned that Ruby has a sore mouth and is struggling to feed. Evie examines Ruby's mouth, which is coated with white spots, and she diagnoses oral thrush. Evie decides to prescribe nystatin oral suspension for Ruby, despite the fact that it is not licensed for use in neonates for the treatment of thrush. Evie has given careful consideration to this and has based her decision on the fact that there is no suitable alternative. Evie is knowledgeable about this well-established medicine and aware that it is not absorbed systemically. She is conscious that she must accept medico-legal responsibility for this, but is confident that she can justify her actions. She feels competent in her ability to diagnose oral thrush and prescribe the nystatin off-label.

Off-label medication

As mentioned above, sometimes a medicine is prescribed for a use that is outside the terms and conditions of its licence (off-label). It is not illegal for doctors to prescribe off-label, and there are a number of circumstances in which nurse independent prescribers may prescribe licensed medicines for a purpose for which they are not licensed, especially when prescribing for children. However, in order to do so they must have ensured that the following conditions apply:

- that the medicine would serve the child's needs better than an appropriately licensed alternative;
- that there is sufficient evidence and/or experience in using the medicine to demonstrate its safety and efficacy;
- if the manufacturer's information leaflet is of limited help, the necessary information has been sought from another source;
- the prescriber has explained to the child and family the reasons why the medicine is not licensed for the proposed use;
- clear and accurate records have been made of the medicine prescribed and the reason for prescribing off-label medicine.

The following activity will help you to identify unlicensed and off-label drugs.

Activity 2.3   *Critical thinking*

Look up the following drugs in the *British National Formulary for Children* and identify their licensed use:

- lansoprazole
- fluoxetine
- nystatin
- caffeine.

Now look up some of the drugs commonly used in your area of practice. Are you surprised at your findings?

Outline answers are provided at the end of the chapter.

Independent nurse prescribing

The Medicinal Products: Prescription by Nurses Act became law in 1992. Amendments to the Medicines Act were made in 1994 and amendments to the pharmaceutical regulations were made to allow pharmacists to dispense medicines prescribed by nurses. Health visitors and community nurses who had recorded their additional nurse prescribing qualification with the NMC were allowed to prescribe from the *Nurse Prescriber's Formulary* (now named the *Nurse Prescribers' Formulary for Community Practitioners* (NPF) (BMA/RPS, 2009)). The majority of the drugs in the formulary were not POMs, but such products as dressings, urinary catheters, stoma care products, scabies and head lice treatments and skin preparations.

Extended formulary nurse prescribing was introduced in 2002, allowing registered nurses and midwives with additional training to prescribe from the NPF. This formulary included more than 120 POMs to be prescribed for specific conditions. It was revised in 2006 to include medicines for emergency care and certain controlled drugs for specific conditions.

Legislation in May 2006 allowed independent prescribing from a full formulary (excluding most controlled drugs) and the *Nurse Prescribers' Extended Formulary* no longer exists. Extended formulary nurse prescribers became nurse independent prescribers, who can prescribe within their area of competence, if agreed by their employer.

Prescribing for children

Only those nurses who have relevant knowledge, competence, skills and experience in nursing children should prescribe for children (NMC, 2006). Anyone prescribing for children in, for example, walk-in centres, primary care and general practice must only do so within their competence or level of expertise. Otherwise they should refer to another prescriber.

Patient group directions

Patient group directions (PGDs) were introduced in 2000 to replace the group protocols, which were thought perhaps to be breaching the law. Amendments to Medicines Act legislation allow for some healthcare professionals to supply or administer medicines in accordance with PGDs.

A PGD is a written direction relating to the sale or supply and administration of a prescription-only medicine (POM) to patients generally, and is signed by a doctor (or dentist) and pharmacist. Ideally, the decision to prescribe is made by a specific prescriber for a specific individual patient. PGDs should only be considered where they would benefit patient care without compromising patient safety in any way. A senior representative of all the healthcare professionals involved, such as doctors and pharmacists, and the professional group expected to supply or administer the medicine under the direction, should be involved in the decision-making process. For example, a registered nurse working in a walk-in centre would be able to supply and administer a salbutamol inhaler to a child without the need for a prescription or an instruction from a prescriber. A PGD would allow the supply and administration of the salbutamol if the child fell into the group defined in the PGD. Using a PGD is not a form of prescribing and registered nurses require no additional formal qualification. It is usual practice for nurses to have training by their employer before being considered competent to use a PGD.

The law states that only a registered nurse may supply and administer a PGD; it cannot be delegated to any other person, including student nurses.

PGDs must contain the following information to be valid:

- the period during which the PGD is effective (PGDs should be reviewed at least every two years);
- the description or class of the POM to which the PGD relates;
- the specific clinical situation that the described POM or class may be used to treat;
- the clinical criteria under which a patient is eligible for treatment;
- whether any specific patients are excluded from treatment under the PGD;
- any circumstances for which further advice should be sought from a doctor;
- any restrictions on the quantity of medicine that may be sold or supplied on any occasion;
- the pharmaceutical forms in which the POM is to be administered;
- the applicable dosage or maximum dosage;
- the route of administration;
- the frequency of administration;
- the minimum or maximum period of administration;
- relevant warnings, including potential adverse reactions;
- follow-up action to take in any circumstances;
- arrangements for referral for medical advice;
- details of the records to be kept.

Persons permitted to supply or administer a PGD under the Regulations are the following *registered* professionals:

- nurses;
- midwives;

- pharmacists;
- paramedics or individuals holding a certificate of proficiency in paramedic skills issued by, or with approval of, the Secretary of State;
- dietitians;
- occupational therapists;
- radiographers;
- physiotherapists;
- optometrists;
- chiropodists;
- orthoptists;
- speech and language therapists;
- orthotists and prosthetists.

Some CDs can be supplied and administered by registered nurses in accordance with a PGD under Misuse of Drugs legislation.

Activity 2.4   *Decision-making*

You are working in a walk-in centre and have been delegated by the registered nurse on shift with you to administer 500mg of paracetamol to a 14-year-old child who the registered nurse has checked under a PGD.

- What should you do?

An outline answer is provided at the end of the chapter.

Supplementary prescribing

Supplementary prescribing is a voluntary partnership between an independent prescriber (who must be a doctor or dentist) and a supplementary prescriber, to implement an agreed patient-specific clinical management plan (CMP), with the patient's agreement.

Supplementary prescribers can prescribe CDs as part of the agreed clinical management plan, as long as the supplementary prescriber is working within his or her level of competence.

Prescribing a POM as a supplementary prescriber outside a CMP constitutes a criminal offence. To prescribe a non-POM outside the agreement of a CMP, the registrant would be subject to both disciplinary proceedings by their employer and referral to the NMC, should a charge of professional misconduct follow.

Registered nurses must only ever prescribe within their level of competence. Where they lack competence, the patient should be referred back to a doctor or dentist.

Safety issues

The following section will begin by looking at the law in relation to the supervision, management and use of controlled drugs. It will then discuss other aspects of safety in medicines management.

The Controlled Drugs (Supervision of Management and Use) Regulations 2006

These regulations require NHS and independent healthcare organisations to appoint an accountable officer whose duties and responsibilities are to improve the management and use of CDs. The regulations also require the individual organisations to cooperate with each other and to share information and concerns about the management of CDs, and to set out arrangements relating to powers of entry and inspection.

The Health Act 2006

The Health Act 2006 requires healthcare organisations and independent hospitals to appoint an accountable officer. Responsible bodies such as healthcare organisations, professional regulatory bodies and police forces have a duty of collaboration to share intelligence on CD issues. The Act provides for powers of entry and inspection for the police and other nominated personnel in order to inspect stocks and records of CDs.

Child safety is considered to be a very important issue within medicines management. This is due to the number of children who accidentally ingest medicines and are poisoned every year, some fatally. There has been various legislation passed in the UK in order to prevent this from happening.

The Medicines (Child Safety) Regulations 2003

These Regulations provide guidelines to ensure that medicines are packaged in containers that children cannot easily open. A child-resistant package is one that is difficult for young children to open and thereby gain access to the contents, but not difficult for adults to use. Exemptions to the requirement to package in child-resistant containers apply to effervescent products and those products packaged in sealed unit dose containers such as sachets. Tablets in dispersible form (such as dispersible aspirin) are not exempt. There are statutory requirements for medicines containing aspirin, paracetamol and more than 24mg of iron to be sold in packaging that is shown to be child-resistant. Iron is particularly harmful to young children, and the amount of iron contained in children's and adult vitamins can be enough to kill a child if taken in excessive amounts.

All methadone should be dispensed in a child-resistant container when prescribed for home consumption, and it should be stored in a safe, locked location. Methadone users should be made aware of the particular risks to children, especially if they have children at home or if children visit their home.

Product labels

In order to promote the safety of medicines there are regulations that ensure they are correctly labelled and easily identifiable.

European Union directives issued in 1992 require specific information to be included on both the outer packaging of drugs and the drug label. You will notice that drug packaging is labelled with the proprietary name and the recommended International Nonproprietary Name (rINN) or generic name. For example, paracetamol is the generic or rINN name, whereas the proprietary or brand name could be Calpol, Medinol, Panadol or Disprol. It is very important you are aware of this, as many parents will not realise that medicines they have been administering to their children, under brand names such as Calpol, actually contain paracetamol. This can lead to over-administration when using two over-the-counter (OTC) products containing paracetamol.

The information on the product label must be clear and legible. Labels are designed to meet the needs of pharmacists, patients, doctors and nurses, so they contain various different kinds of information. This includes having appropriate warnings and instructions on labels and leaflets supplied with medicines. Packs conforming to European Union directives are called 'patient packs' and are ready-to-dispense packs that always contain a 'patient information leaflet' (PIL) supplied by the pharmaceutical company.

Patient information leaflets

Manufacturers must by law provide a PIL within the medicine packaging, and this information is often highly valued by patients. Children and families have to make decisions about medicines and these should be informed decisions.

However carefully medicine is prescribed and provided to children, there is no guarantee it will be taken as advised. Also, the manufacturer's PIL will only cover the licensed use of the medicine. Therefore, when a medicine is being used outside its product licence you may need to advise the child and family that some of the information in the leaflet may not be applicable to the child's treatment.

Children and young people need to be given information about their medicines in the same way that adults are. However, PILs are designed for adults and are not aimed at children. It is good practice to give enough information as possible to the child and family. This information should include the proposed course of treatment, and any known serious or common side effects of, or adverse reactions to, the medicine. Ideally, the unsuitable advice in the PIL should be identified and the child and family offered reassurance about the correct use of the medicine in the context of the child's condition.

The following scenario highlights how easy it is for parents to over-administer over-the-counter paracetamol.

Scenario

Simon is a paediatric nurse practitioner in a paediatric accident and emergency department. He has just assessed 2-year-old Lucy, who has had a minor head injury, and is discharging her home, giving her mother advice on what to do following head injury. Simon also advises Lucy's mother that it is possible that Lucy might have a mild headache and that some paracetamol or ibuprofen might help this. Lucy's mother says that she will

continued overleaf . . .

continued . . .

> buy some paracetamol from the supermarket to give to her. Simon decides to check if Lucy's mum is giving her any other medicines, to which she replies, 'Just a spoon of Calpol at bedtime to help her sleep'. Simon then explains to Lucy's mum that Calpol, Disprol and Tixymol are all brand names for paracetamol, and that there is no need for her to buy more. He advises Lucy's mum that it is important to be careful not to give Lucy too much paracetamol, as often cold remedies will also contain amounts of the drug. He also stresses to Lucy's mum that paracetamol (Calpol) should be used for the management of pain or fever and it is not useful in helping children to sleep.
>
> Simon has found from experience that parents are often not aware that OTC children's medicines such as Disprol contain paracetamol.

The Royal College of Paediatrics and Child Health produced a leaflet that can be given to parents to support verbal information on the use of unlicensed medicines in children (RCPCH, 2000).

Consent

As a nurse you must act in accordance with the NMC *Code* (2008) in relation to consent.

- You must ensure that you gain consent before you begin any treatment or care.
- You must respect and support people's rights to accept or decline treatment and care.
- You must uphold people's rights to be fully involved in decisions about their care.

Consent in children and young people is a very complex area, but you must be sure to gain consent before administering any medication to a child. If children are competent to give consent for themselves, you should seek consent directly from them.

Young people 16 and 17 years old

Young people aged 16 and 17 years are able by law to consent to their own treatment in the same way as adults can. It is not necessary to obtain the consent of the parent or guardian of a 16 or 17 year old, or to inform them if the young person agrees to treatment. It is, however, considered good practice to encourage these 'competent children' to involve their parents in the decision making.

If a young person less than 18 years old finds it too difficult to decide for themselves, or does not feel they understand enough, their parents or guardian may give consent on their behalf. Also, until a young person reaches the age of 18 years, the parents may override the refusal of their child to consent to treatment. It is exceptional for these disagreements to occur, but when they do it may be necessary for a court to decide whether the treatment should go ahead.

There will be certain medicines available over the counter that older children may purchase and use without adult supervision. There is no legal age limit for buying OTC medicines. It is up to the discretion of the pharmacist to decide to sell or refuse a medicine to a child or young person.

When a medicine is not licensed for use in children of their age, the pharmacist must not sell the medicine to them for their own use. There are no guidelines from the MHRA or the Royal Pharmaceutical Society (RPS) on this issue (NHS Choices, 2010).

Children under 16 years

Children and young people under the age of 16 years are not automatically presumed by law to be competent to make their own decisions about healthcare. The right to consent to treatment rests with the child's parents or guardian, unless the child under 16 years is considered to have *sufficient understanding and intelligence to enable him or her to understand fully what is proposed* (Lord Scarman in *Gillick* v *West Norfolk and Wisbech Area HA* (1986)). This is known as 'Gillick competence', and means there is no specific age at which a child becomes competent to consent to treatment; it depends on the seriousness and complexity of the proposed treatment. For example, a child of 13 or 14 may be competent to consent to taking paracetamol for pain relief, but may not be competent to consent to life-threatening cardiac surgery (although they should still be involved in the decision making).

Activity 2.5 — *Critical thinking*

You are working as a school nurse and are running an immunisation clinic administering HPV vaccinations to protect against cervical cancer. Fiona, who is 14 years old, wants to have the vaccination but her parents would rather she did not.

- Is Fiona able to consent for herself?
- What should you do in this situation?

Outline answers are provided at the end of the chapter.

Activity 2.6 — *Critical thinking*

Anya is 15 years old and refuses to have chemotherapy because she does not wish to suffer the side effects of nausea and hair loss, and believes she can get better herself without it. She seems to be competent to make up her own mind about this decision and fully understands the implications of refusing treatment. Her parents disagree with her decision and want to consent to the treatment.

- What should and can happen in Anya's case?
- What do you think would be the best solution to Anya's case?

Outline answers are provided at the end of the chapter.

Confidentiality

The NMC *Code* (2008) states that you must respect people's rights to confidentiality, and that children and young people are entitled to the same rights to confidentiality as adults. This applies to medicines management as much as any other area of nursing care.

As a nurse, you must ensure that children and young people are informed about how and why information is shared between people providing their care. However, if you believe the child or young person may be at risk of harm, you must then disclose information in line with the law of the country in which you are practising.

Research involving children

In order to improve medical care of children, research involving children is essential, but it must be conducted in an ethical manner. Children are unique as a research group, as they are the only client group in British law who may have other individuals such as parents consenting on their behalf. Research should only be undertaken on children if it is not possible to undertake the research on adults with comparable results.

Drug metabolism is different in children from that in adults, and adverse events may occur that are not predictable from adult trials. All research proposals involving children should be submitted for approval by a research ethics committee. Consent should be obtained from the child or parent as appropriate. Where parental consent is obtained to include the child in research, the agreement of the child should also be requested by the researchers if the child is of school age (RCPCH, 2000). It is not illegal or necessarily considered unethical to conduct a research procedure that is not intended to directly benefit the child subject.

The following activities will help you to consider the ethical implications of clinical trials involving children.

Activity 2.7   *Reflection*

Bringing a new drug on to the market is a costly process and can cost millions of pounds, most of the cost being towards the funding of clinical trials. Many Western drug companies, British included, are moving their clinical trials to poorer countries such as India and China, where costs are greatly reduced.

- How do you feel about clinical trials being conducted on children in India and China in order to benefit Western children?

An outline answer is provided at the end of the chapter.

Activity 2.8   *Evidence-based practice and research*

In October 2009, families in the UK were asked to take part in the trials for swine flu (Influenza H1N1) vaccine. The trials were to determine which of two swine flu vaccines already tested in adults was the most effective in children aged between 6 months and 12 years. The children would receive two doses of a swine flu vaccine three weeks apart and a blood sample of 6 to 10mL would be taken three weeks after the second vaccine in order to assess the efficacy. A total of 1,000 children were asked to participate in this study, 500 aged 6 months to 3 years and 500 aged 3 years to 12 years (**www.swineflutrial.org/ swineflu_screen_suht.html**).

- What do you think were some of the ethical considerations when the study was approved by the Oxfordshire Research Ethics Committee and the MHRA?

An outline answer is provided at the end of the chapter.

Chapter summary

This chapter has outlined the legal frameworks in relation to safe administration of medicines in practice. You should now have some knowledge and understanding of the background to the law and to your practice, including the more recent changes such as non-medical prescribing. You should also have an understanding of the law in relation to patient group directions and the supply and administration of medicines. Ethical issues and consent in relation to medicines and children have been considered and you have reflected on potential scenarios.

Activities: brief outline answers

Activity 2.1 Identifying POMs (page 43)

- Amoxicillin: this is a prescription-only medicine, so you will find the PoM symbol next to the name in the BNF.
- Chlorphenamine maleate: you will find that, in the form of an injection, it is a PoM, but this restriction does not apply when administration is for saving life in an emergency. In tablet and syrup form it is a pharmacy (P) medicine.
- Hydrocortisone: again, this is a PoM dependent on the form and strength. It can be bought over the counter as a P drug in its mildest form for specific conditions such as insect bites, irritant dermatitis and mild to moderate eczema in children over 10 years.

Activity 2.2 Schedules of controlled drugs (page 46)

- phentermine – Schedule 3
- lorazepam – Schedule 4, part I
- pethidine – Schedule 2
- fentanyl – Schedule 2

Activity 2.3 Licensed uses of drugs (page 53)

If you look up the generic name in the BNF, you will find the **licensed use** stated underneath **cautions** and **side effects**.

• Lansoprazole is not licensed for use in children.
• Fluoxetine is not licensed for use in children.
• Nystatin suspension is not licensed for use in neonates; the suspension is licensed for prophylaxis in neonates as a once daily dose; tablets are not licensed for use in children (age range not specified by manufacturer). This is interesting, as you may find many neonates prescribed nystatin for oral thrush. A young child prescribed nystatin tablets has died from asphyxiation following accidental inhalation.
• Caffeine – no licensed product is available (this is an unlicensed drug).

Activity 2.4 Patient group directions (page 55)

You should not accept the delegated task from the registered nurse who is responsible for administering the drug herself under a PGD.

The law states that only a registered nurse may supply and administer a PGD, so this cannot be delegated to any other person, including student nurses.

Activity 2.5 Consent of children under 16 years (page 59)

As the school nurse, you should try to involve Fiona's parents in the decision making, and could offer to talk to them, perhaps over the telephone, and discuss the benefits of the vaccination. Even though Fiona is under the age of 16 years, if you have assessed her as being 'Gillick competent', that is, you feel she fully understands what is involved in having the vaccination, she can consent for herself even without her parents' agreement. The vaccination can legally go ahead, although it is always better to gain the agreement of the parents.

Activity 2.6 Consent of a child to chemotherapy (page 59)

By law, Anya's parents can override her refusal to treatment. However, it would be very unfair to betray Anya's trust and enforce treatment. But if Anya is not treated, the implications would be very serious. A decision should be made to ask a court to decide what is in Anya's 'best interests'. It is likely the court will decide that Anya should have the treatment, which she may find easier to accept as it has not been forced on her by those people closely involved with her.

Activity 2.7 Research involving children (page 60)

Research involving children and young people should only be conducted where the research is important for the health and well-being of children. Research that is not intended to directly to benefit the child subject is not necessarily unethical. All proposals involving research on children must be submitted to a research ethics committee. The Declaration of Helsinki includes recommendations where children are research subjects in relation to informed consent.

When the child is unable to consent for themselves, permission from the responsible family member should be sought in accordance with national legislation. It is possible that poor and uneducated parents do not understand the full implications of volunteering their children for drug trials. Parents may be happy to volunteer their children for altruistic reasons or for a small payment for their expenses. They may feel that being included in a clinical trial is better than no healthcare at all.

Are Western companies exploiting these parents and children to test new medicines, when it is unlikely that they will be able to afford to buy them once they are licensed and marketed? Why should drugs that have not been proved safe in their country of origin be tested on children in poorer countries?

Activity 2.8 Swine flu trials (page 61)

There are many questions that would have been considered by the ethics committee when approving these clinical trials. Assessment of the potential benefit of the trials would have included how severe the problem is and how would the knowledge gained be used. Given the magnitude of swine flu and its severity for the UK population, it would have been considered a huge benefit for many children. The research would have been considered to be very likely to achieve its aims, and the children taking part would themselves benefit by receiving the vaccine and having their immunity established, therefore potentially protecting them from serious illness. The other benefits of the research would be the potential financial saving to the UK, preventing the cost of serious illness, and being able to choose the most cost-effective vaccine.

Assessment of the potential harm of the trials would consider how intrusive the research is. The vaccinations the children would potentially be receiving anyway, despite the trials, were made readily available. Taking of a blood sample can be painful and distressing, particularly for younger children who are not able to consent for themselves. Children's responses to interventions such as phlebotomy are varied and unpredictable. A procedure that does not bother one child may cause severe distress in another. It could be argued that a procedure such as this is inappropriate if the child is unlikely to benefit from the experience. The pain and distress and the memory of it might cause more than minimal harm. Should parents be allowed to consent to their babies experiencing the pain of taking blood in order to benefit other infants? Recommendations would be made to ensure that all steps are taken to reduce the amount of pain and distress to a minimum by using local anaesthetic cream and distraction, for example.

Might the adverse effects be brief or long lasting? The ethics committee would seem to have enough confidence in the information gained about the vaccine from adults to risk trials with children. But how do we know about the long-term effects if the vaccine is newly produced? It would be considered a positive point that the children to be included in the study were without medical problems, so the researchers were not relying on children who already have many problems. There would be no harm from withholding treatment as the trials were between two vaccines and not with a placebo, so all children would benefit from this.

Other considerations you may have thought about include the inconvenience to the family, such as the three clinic visits (families were reimbursed £10 for this). What support and follow-up were the families offered? What about the size of the study – were enough children involved to make a statistically valid sample, allowing for withdrawals from the study? Or was the planned number of children unnecessarily too high?

You may have thought of many more ethical considerations about this study; perhaps you could debate these issues with some colleagues.

Further reading

Department of Health (DH) (2001) *Consent – What You Have a Right to Expect: A guide for children and young people.* London: Department of Health.

This document tells children and young people how consent is asked for and given, what they need to know before giving consent, how old they have to be, whether their parents should be involved, when other people can give consent for them, and what to do if they are asked to take part in research. It is available on the department's website at **www.dh.gov.uk**.

Department of Health (DH) (2001) *Seeking Consent: Working with children.* London: Department of Health.

This explains who can give consent and covers some more complex situations. It is available on the department's website at **www.dh.gov.uk**.

Department of Health (DH) (2002) *Safeguarding Children in Whom Illness is Fabricated or Induced.* London: Department of Health.

This is supplementary guidance to *Working Together to Safeguard Children* and is available on the department's website at **www.dh.gov.uk**.

Nursing and Midwifery Council (NMC) (2006) *Standards of Proficiency for Nurse and Midwifery Prescribers.* London: NMC.

This provides the standards of conduct that nurses and midwives are required to meet in their practice as registered nurse prescribes and is available at the 'Publications' section of the Council's website at **www.nmc-uk.org**.

Useful websites

http://mcrn.org.uk

The National Institute for Health Research Medicines for Children Research Network is funded by the Department of Health and works to improve the UK's clinical research environment and maximise the development of safe and effective medicines and formulations for children.

www.homeoffice.gov.uk/documents

A list of drugs controlled under the misuse of drugs legislation, including their classification under both the Misuse of Drugs Act 1971 and the Misuse of Drugs Regulations 2001, is available on this Home Office website.

www.medicinesforchildren.org.uk/index.php

The Medicines for Children website provides information leaflets specifically about the use of medicines in children. They are written for parents and carers but may also be suitable for older children.

www.mhra.gov.uk/Publications/PublicAssessmentReports/PublicAssessmentReportsfor herbalmedicines/index.htm

The Medicines and Healthcare products Regulatory Agency (MHRA) provides Public Assessment Reports for traditional herbal medicines.

www.nes.scot.nhs.uk/pharmacy/paediatrics/Key%20documents/OLDER%20CHILDREN. PDF

This is the Royal College of Paediatrics and Child Health Medicines for Children Information for older children.

www.nhs.uk/Pages/HomePage.aspx

This NHS Choices website provides further information on fabricated or induced illness.

www.npci.org.uk/cd/public/legislation.php

The NHS National Prescribing Centre website supports the safe and effective use of controlled drugs within England. It contains resources and information about the management and prescribing of controlled drugs. The website gives an overview of the legislation of controlled drugs with links to further websites.

www.legislation.gov.uksi/2001/3998/contents/made

This Office for Public Sector Information web page contains the Misuse of Drugs Regulations 2001.

www.rcpch.ac.uk

The Royal College of Paediatrics and Child Health is responsible for the training and examination of paediatricians in the UK. It also undertakes research and policy generation.

Chapter 3
Holistic care and treatment options in children's nursing

NMC Standards for Pre-registration Nursing Education

This chapter will address the following competencies:

Domain 1: Professional values
2. All nurses must practise in a holistic, non-judgmental, caring and sensitive manner that avoids assumptions; supports social inclusion; recognises and respects individual choice; and acknowledges diversity. Where necessary, they must challenge inequality, discrimination and exclusion from access to care.
5. All nurses must fully understand the nurse's various roles, responsibilities and functions, and adapt their practice to meet the changing needs of people, groups, communities and populations.
6. All nurses must understand the roles and responsibilities of other health and social care professionals, and seek to work with them collaboratively for the benefit of all who need care.

NMC Essential Skills Clusters

This chapter will address the following ESCs:

Cluster: Medicines management
35. People can trust the newly registered graduate nurse to work as part of a team to offer holistic care and a range of treatment options of which medicines may form a part.

By the second progression point:
1. Demonstrates awareness of a range of commonly recognised approaches to managing symptoms, for example relaxation, distraction and lifestyle advice.
2. Discusses referral options.

By entry to the register:
3. Works confidently as part of the team and, where relevant, as leader of the team to develop treatment options and choices with the person receiving care and their carers.
4. Questions, critically appraises, takes into account ethical considerations and the preferences of the person receiving care and uses evidence to support an argument in determining when medicines may or may not be an appropriate choice of treatment.

continued overleaf . . .

continued . . . •••

42. People can trust the newly registered graduate nurse to demonstrate understanding and knowledge to supply and administer via a patient group direction.

By the second progression point:
1. Demonstrates knowledge of what a patient group direction is and who can use them.

Chapter aims

By the end of this chapter, you should be able to:

- appreciate the role of other health professionals in the administration of medicines;
- demonstrate an awareness of the use of over-the-counter medicines;
- appreciate the importance of health promotion and lifestyle advice in relation to medicines management;
- understand the principles of holistic care;
- consider other treatment options in place of medicines, or as adjuvants to medicines for the management of illness.

Case study

Jenny was working as a nurse in primary care, in a walk-in medical centre. One evening she was surprised to encounter a parent who had driven three miles at seven o'clock in the evening, to wait in the walk-in centre and to be assessed by a busy nurse, in order to receive her 'free bottle of paracetamol'. The parent felt she was entitled to this; she said her GP always wrote a paracetamol prescription for her. She didn't want a diagnosis or any advice, as she knew her child had a minor childhood illness (hand, foot and mouth disease), which he had contracted from nursery. She knew how to manage the symptoms.

Jenny refused her a 'free bottle' and advised her that she could buy paracetamol from a 24-hour supermarket and pharmacy.

Why did Jenny advise the parent to buy her own over-the-counter medicine? One of the nurse's tasks is to discourage dependent behaviour on the NHS budget (bearing in mind both the cost of a prescription and a consultation) and to promote independence in patients. It is the responsibility of healthcare professionals to give information and advice on access to medicines and the appropriate self-management of illness. It would have been acceptable to have given a prescription if it was likely the parent could not afford to buy the medicine.

Introduction

Directing parents towards self-care and management of their child's minor ailments and illness is essential in order to ensure that parents are able to take control of their child's health and well-being. Self-care is not about expecting parents to manage alone, but empowering parents through providing the information they need to make healthy lifestyle choices, take control and feel more confident in parenting and childcare.

The children's nurse needs to be aware of some of the common over-the-counter (OTC) medications and other treatment options available to parents, in order to give sound advice about their safety and efficacy. This chapter will give a brief overview of some of the more commonly used treatment options, but is by no means inclusive. As a registered children's nurse it is essential that you work as part of a team offering holistic care and a range of treatment options to the child and family, and medicines will form a part of that range.

The chapter starts by giving an overview of the roles and responsibilities of some other healthcare professionals in the team, so that you are prepared for working together and can make appropriate referrals.

Providing lifestyle advice to children and families is an essential part of the nurse's role, helping parents to make healthy choices for themselves and their children. This chapter can only touch on some basic principles of lifestyle advice, but will direct you towards further resources on lifestyle available to parents and health professionals. Living a healthy lifestyle is an important part of self-care for everyone, and in the long term will reduce dependency on healthcare and the increasing use of medicines in society. From my experience, a class of student nurses will usually give the answer 'administer analgesia' in response to the question of how would they manage a child's pain. Very few would consider other alternatives, such as massage, imagery, aromatherapy or distraction, unless the child was undergoing a specific procedure. Yet these are the very responses that come naturally to a parent, although it may take the form of 'rub it better', 'let's have a cuddle' or 'never mind, let's read a nice story'. It is part of the children's nurse's role to offer alternative treatment options and apply them to practice, instead of just reaching for the medicine pot.

The chapter will discuss some of the complementary and alternative medicines (CAMs) and therapies and the principles of holistic care and how that should influence our practice.

The roles and responsibilities of other healthcare professionals

Prescribers

Due to the recent changes in the law, the prescriber could be a doctor, pharmacist, nurse or allied health professional. The prescriber remains responsible for the decision making after consultation with the child and family as to whether a medicine or another treatment option is the best choice

and family. The prescriber should also be responsible for educating the child and
eir medicines and their expected benefits and side effects. The prescriber should
child and family with the reasons why one particular treatment option has been
another.

Pharmacists

Pharmacists both in a hospital and in the community have an important role in the safe and
appropriate use of medicines for children and young people. Some hospital pharmacists working
within multidisciplinary teams have specialist knowledge of areas such as neonatal and paediatric
pharmacy, or may have specialised in areas such as intensive care, paediatric oncology, or renal
or cardiac services. Hospital pharmacists are able to give advice on the management of medicines
and ensure that medicines are appropriate for the child's age, development and clinical condition.
Pharmacists are also able to liaise with community services in order to ensure that arrangements
are made for the continuation of the child's care following discharge. The pharmacist will also
provide information on the efficacy and cost of different medicines.

Community pharmacists are involved in ensuring that policies are in place for the safe and
effective use of medicines across the Primary Care Trust (PCT) by engaging in the commissioning
of services for children and influencing the prescribing patterns of general practitioners. This
would include developing shared care guidelines across primary, secondary and tertiary care.
Community pharmacists have a health promotion role in the provision of healthy lifestyle advice,
such as on healthy eating, exercise, lowering alcohol intake and stopping smoking. Some community pharmacists will also provide minor illness advice, and pharmacists who have completed
the independent prescribing qualification are able to prescribe medicines for children as long as
it is within their professional and clinical competence.

Young people may access community pharmacists for emergency hormonal contraception. The
pharmacist is subject to the RPS's Code of Ethics in relation to confidentiality when providing
these services. The pharmacist is in a key position to advise parents on OTC preparations and
the self-administration of medicines for children.

Physiotherapists

The role of the physiotherapist is to assess and manage children and young people with movement disorders, disabilities or illness, working in close partnership with families and the multi-
disciplinary team. They provide advice, support and physical interventions to children and
families, to enable children to meet their full potential. Physiotherapists have been administering
medicines under patient specific directions (PSDs) for injection therapy since the 1990s. Since
2000 they have been able to supply and administer medicines to children under PGDs (see
Chapter 2, pages 54–5) and if they have completed the relevant training as supplementary
prescribers. Supplementary prescribing is being increasingly used by physiotherapists to prescribe
a wide range of medicines for the management of musculoskeletal, respiratory and neurological
conditions and for pain management.

Dietitians

Dietitians assess, give advice about and manage the care of children with disorders where dietary intervention and nutritional support is required. They are able to see children with a wide range of disorders, such as delayed growth, increased calorie requirement and poor oral intake. Dietitians are able to supply and administer medicines to children under PSDs and PGDs for nutritional support for conditions such as cystic fibrosis, diabetes and gastric disorders. They are able to give advice to other health professionals on appropriate prescriptions, such as feed supplements for the management of nutritional status. Children who are unable to eat and drink and who need enteral (tube feeding) or parenteral (intravenous) nutrition should be referred to the dietitian. Dietitians are able to prepare special therapeutic feeds and diets for infants and children. Their health education role includes giving expert advice on nutritional matters and developing written resources for families and healthcare professionals.

Radiographers

Diagnostic radiographers produce images of organs, limbs and other body parts to enable doctors (and other advanced practitioners) to make diagnoses. Therapeutic radiographers use high-energy radiation to treat cancer. Radiographers are able to supply and administer medicines under PSDs and PGDs, and if they have completed the relevant training as supplementary prescribers. Therapeutic radiographers are able to use PGDs and PSDs to manage pain and the side effects of radiotherapy. Diagnostic radiographers are able, under supplementary prescribing, to administer analgesics or anti-emetics before, during or after procedures. Most radiographic contrast agents are prescribed under PGDs or PSDs.

Speech and language therapists

Speech and language therapists (SLTs) assess children who may have speech and language difficulties, or eating and drinking difficulties. They work closely with the child and family, healthcare professionals, and education and social services in order to meet the child's needs. SLTs are able to supply and administer medicines to children under PGDs and PSDs in order to assist procedures such as video fluoroscopy. The SLT is able to play a key role in the assessment and recommendation of those borderline substances such as thickened feeds for infants and children with gastroesophageal reflux.

Occupational therapists

The occupational therapist (OT) works with children who have difficulties with the practical and social skills necessary for everyday life. The aim of the OT is to enable children to be physically, socially and psychologically independent. The OT is able to supply and administer medicines to children under PGDs. The OT is more likely to prescribe equipment to children (such as splints, cutlery or pencil grips) to prevent deformities and make tasks easier.

Play specialists

Play specialists work closely with the multidisciplinary team to lead playful activities with children and use play as a therapeutic tool. The play specialist uses an understanding of child development to plan play activities to help children cope with pain, anxiety and fear. The play specialist is able to spend time with a child, getting to know them better, and can explain worrying procedures with the use of dolls, books and videos. The play specialist can help a child cope with a painful or difficult procedure through the use of distraction therapy.

Optometrists

Optometrists diagnose and treat vision problems in children. All children should be assessed by an optometrist before they start school and start learning to read. The earlier a vision problem is detected, the more chance there is of successful treatment. Optometrist prescribers can prescribe any licensed medicine for conditions connected with the eye that they are competent to treat.

The following scenario is useful in demonstrating the roles of other health professionals in medicines management.

Scenario

Six-year-old Martha has partial-thickness burns to her hands and arms, and gets very distressed during her physiotherapy sessions and when she has her wound dressings changed. Judy, the nurse caring for Martha, and the physiotherapist discussed this problem with the pharmacist, who suggested the use of Entonox during the procedures. Entonox is a mixture of inhaled nitrous oxide and oxygen and is a useful analgesic for painful procedures. Martha was old enough to self-regulate the Entonox using a demand valve, which reduced her fear and gave her some control over the situation. Judy also arranged for the play specialist to be present during the dressing changes who used play as a form of distraction. The OT was also involved in Martha's care and assessed Martha for hand splints to prevent contractures and deformities of her hands and arms. The OT liaised with the nurses and the doctor who prescribed her analgesia to ensure that Martha was pain free when wearing the splints and tolerated them better.

Over-the-counter preparations

Parents will always make personal choices regarding medicines they self-administer to their children, and many over-the-counter (OTC) preparations are available to them. OTC preparations are available to parents at their local high-street pharmacies or at local supermarkets, and some forms of therapy, such as chamomile and ginseng, at local health food shops. Parents will be encouraged to purchase and make use of these products through advertisements on television, in magazines and through discussions with other parents and friends and relatives. Parents' decisions will also be influenced by the marketing ploys used in supermarkets frequented by parents, such as display, packaging and special offers. All these products are available without a prescription and many without the supervision of a pharmacist. Parents will use these products to manage a wide range of minor illnesses and ailments, such as coughs and upper respiratory tract infections, hayfever, constipation, colic, diarrhoea, travel sickness, mild pain, musculoskeletal problems and many others. It is very much the focus of healthcare today to encourage self-care in patients, as this is a significant factor in reducing costs to the health service. However, this must be carefully balanced with good health education and medicines advice, in order to ensure patients' safety. The children's nurse should encourage self-care and health promotion, but also offer advice to parents on the appropriate use of OTC products and the potential problems.

One of the most worrying aspects of self-care in children, young babies in particular, is that parents may fail to recognise a seriously unwell child until it is too late for successful medical intervention. The signs and symptoms of more serious illnesses, such as meningitis, can be similar to those of other more common illnesses, such as flu. For this reason, voluntary organisations such as the Meningitis Trust produce symptom cards, advising parents to trust their instincts and get medical help immediately. OTC preparations such as paracetamol carry warnings for parents to seek out medical advice if their child's fever persists for more than three days.

The following scenario demonstrates how registered nurses can be called upon in different situations to give advice on OTC medicines.

Scenario

Julie is a registered nurse who works for NHS Direct providing telephone advice. It is Monday morning and Julie receives a telephone call from Molly, who has a 13-month-old baby called Jack. Jack has had a cough over the weekend that has disturbed his sleep. Julie completes a full assessment of Jack over the telephone. He is well, has no other symptoms and is feeding normally. Molly would like Julie's advice on what she can buy from her local supermarket pharmacy department to treat his cough and help him sleep better. Julie informs Molly that there is no evidence that cough remedies work in young children and that they can cause side effects. Julie advises Molly not to give Jack any OTC medications but to ensure that he gets plenty to drink. Julie tells Molly that coughs and colds are usually self-limiting conditions that get better by themselves. However, if Jack does not get better after five days, or develops any other worrying symptoms, Molly should again seek advice from a health professional.

Children's over-the-counter cough and cold medicines

The Commission on Human Medicines has recently reviewed the advice on the use of OTC cough medicines in the UK. It is now advised that parents and carers should no longer give OTC cough and cold medicines to children under 6 years. This is because there is no evidence that they work, and they can cause side effects such as allergic reactions, effects on sleep and hallucinations. These medicines will continue to be available for children of 6–12 years, as the risk of side effects is reduced in this age group due to the fact that they weigh more, they get fewer coughs and colds, and the child is able to say if the medicine is making them feel any better. Manufacturers were required to update the packaging and leaflets for cough and cold products for children under 12 years in 2009, in order to improve safety.

You should advise parents to administer these medicines carefully in accordance with the manufacturer's instructions and to always ensure the child does not receive more than the maximum dose. You should also advise parents to review medicines they have in their medicine cupboard regularly, and if they have any they no longer need to take them to their local pharmacy for disposal.

So what should parents do when their child has a cough or cold?

Parents should be advised that coughs and colds are self-limiting conditions and will usually get better by themselves. Parents can administer paracetamol or ibuprofen to reduce their child's temperature, as long as it is administered in accordance with the instructions on the label and they are not giving their child any other products that may contain these ingredients. Ensure that the child gets plenty to drink and is encouraged to rest. Young babies may need smaller, more frequent feeds. Nasal aspirators are advertised to parents to suck mucus from the baby's nostrils before feeds. There are no research trials to show whether these are effective and there are concerns that, if not used correctly, they may do some harm. The NMC *Code* (2008) states that *You must ensure any advice you give is evidence based if you are suggesting healthcare products or services.* Children over 1 year can be offered warm drinks of lemon and honey to help ease the cough (DH, 2009a). You should give health promotion advice to never smoke or allow others to smoke around children. Parents should be advised to seek medical advice if their child is not getting better after four or five days.

The following scenario will demonstrate how you must always be alert to the needs of infants and young children when giving advice.

Scenario

Julie is a registered nurse who works for NHS Direct providing telephone advice. It is Friday evening and Julie receives a telephone call from Kay, who has a 3-month-old baby called Tilly. Kay says that Tilly has had a cough and runny nose for about three days. Kay bought some paracetamol from the local pharmacy and gave Tilly half a teaspoon (60mg) about an hour ago. Kay has called NHS Direct as the paracetamol does not seem to have made Tilly any better and she would like advice on what else she can try. Julie completes a full assessment of Tilly's symptoms over the telephone before offering advice. Julie discovers that Tilly has been off her feeds all day, has a temperature of 40°C, seems listless and has a weak high-pitched cry. Julie decides that the safest course of action is to advise Kay to telephone an ambulance to take Tilly to her local emergency department immediately for further assessment.

Sometimes parents can be unsure as to how serious some symptoms can be and how they require medical help, or when it is appropriate to use OTC medications. Tilly is a very young baby with some quite worrying symptoms that need medical assessment. Like Julie, you should always complete a full assessment of the child's symptoms before giving OTC advice. If you do not, then you could risk a more serious illness being missed and treatment delayed.

Health promotion

Health promotion in children and young people is an important healthcare objective in order to prevent disease in the population and to promote a healthy society (DH, 1996, 2009b). The foundations of future health and well-being are laid down during pregnancy and the early years of life (DH, 2008). This is also a time when parents are particularly receptive to making positive changes to their own and their children's lifestyles.

Children's nurses can have a positive impact on child health and the prevention of disease by using every opportunity to give good health education advice to children and families. This might include encouraging breastfeeding initiation and continuation, vaccination and immunisation advice, healthy eating and increased activity, safety advice and other care that helps to keep children healthy and safe.

Activity 3.1   *Team working*

The aim of Sure Start Children's Centres is to improve outcomes for all children and ensure every child gets the best start in life. They now serve most communities, providing services for children under 5 years, although services vary to suit local need. Take the opportunity on your next community placement to visit the local Sure Start Children's Centre.

- What child and family health services are provided there, such as health screening and health visitor services?
- What alternative treatments are offered there, such as massage, relaxation, aromatherapy?
- How does Sure Start differ from traditional health services?

As the answers are based on your own practice area, there are no answers at the end of the chapter. You might want to write something about your experience of Sure Start in your reflective diary.

The following scenario demonstrates a health promotion activity in relation to medicines management.

Scenario

Lisa is a newly qualified staff nurse on a paediatric cardiology ward. She is discharging baby Oliver, who has been diagnosed with a congenital heart defect. Oliver's take-home medication includes the cardiac glycoside digoxin. Lisa is giving discharge advice to his mother Jennifer. Lisa is aware that Jennifer has another two children at home under the age of four. Lisa feels it is important to reinforce safe storage of medicines advice with Jennifer as digoxin is potentially fatal if accidentally ingested. Lisa gives the following advice about the safety of medicines.

She acknowledges that it is hard to keep account of what children are doing at all times and prevent them getting into mischief. It is important that Jennifer is aware that children have a natural curiosity and it is

continued overleaf . . .

continued . . .

> *possible they will try medicines if they are left lying about. Jennifer should explain the dangers to the children, even though they are very young, as it will help minimise the risk. Jennifer should also explain to her children that they should never take medicine unless it is given to them by a trusted adult and never by themselves. Jennifer should not rely on the child-proof safety caps on the medicine because children can be very clever and learn to open them. It is important that medicines are not kept in the baby bag, but are stored in a high, locked cabinet out of children's reach. Jennifer should throw out any medicine that has expired or is left over.*
>
> *Although the advice might seem very basic and common sense, you cannot assume that all parents will have thought about the safe storage of medicines. It may not be a priority in Jennifer's thoughts, as she is adapting to Jack's needs. Often parents are taken aback when the first indication that their child has acquired another skill is when they have an unintentional injury (such as learning to roll and fall off the couch) or ingest something dangerous (by learning to open the child-proof bottle).*

It is important to signpost families to wider support, such as Sure Start Children's Centres, and to make appropriate referrals to other professionals, such as health visitors and school nurses. Telephone advice is available to parents by calling NHS Direct on 0845 46 47.

Lifestyle: diet, exercise, environment and culture

Diet

What we eat can make a huge difference to our health and well-being. Eating more fruit and vegetables packed with essential vitamins, minerals and fibre may help to reduce the risk of diseases like cancer and heart disease. Children being overweight can lead to health problems such as type 2 diabetes, hypertension, and respiratory disorders and coronary heart disease in later life. The government's Change4Life campaign gives advice to families on cutting back fat in the diet, reducing sugar, choosing five portions of fruit and vegetables per day and giving 'me size meals' to children, in order to promote and maintain health. Families will often turn to healthcare professionals, such as naturopath practitioners, chiropractors, acupuncturists and lay advisers, about specific diets in seeking out cures for illness. Several diets have been recommended and tried for ADHD; severe dietary restriction risks caloric deprivation and nutritional deficiencies, and families should always seek the advice of a dietitian.

Exercise

Research evidence clearly supports the inclusion of regular physical exercise for the prevention of chronic disease and for the improvement of overall health. The numerous health benefits of exercise are dependent on the type, intensity and amount of activity undertaken. Regular exercise is known to improve strength, self-esteem and body image, and has many stress-reducing benefits, which may enhance the immune system. The government's Change4Life health promotion campaign recommends that children need at least 60 minutes of physical activity that gets their heart beating faster than normal every day. Regular exercise helps to burn off calories and prevent children storing up excess body fat, which can lead to cancer, type 2 diabetes and heart disease. Weight-bearing exercise such as skipping, dancing and jumping is known to promote healthy bones and prevent osteoporosis in later life. There is a growing interest in Eastern meditative exercises such as tai chi and yoga, and their potential influence on chronic illnesses such as cancer and asthma. Rest is also vitally important for children, and insufficient sleep appears to contribute to pain and suffering in children with chronic illness.

Environment

Environmental influences on children can be both helpful and stressful. Environmental strategies include the use of light as phototherapy in the treatment of jaundice, vibration in the management of infantile colic (Huhtala et al., 2000) and the use of music to reduce stress (Allen et al., 2001). Skin-to-skin contact is a recommended strategy after birth to encourage mother and infant attachment and bonding (Moore et al., 2007). Other environmental strategies include hot and cold packs for the management of musculoskeletal injury (MacAuley, 2001), transcutaneous electrical nerve stimulation (TENS) for the management of pain (Lander and Fowler-Kerry, 1992) and aromatherapy, which can be helpful in reducing pain and anxiety. Other common sense interventions that rely on individual child preferences include bright or dim lights, and the use of colours, photographs and other types of art, sounds, music and favourite objects to contribute to the child's comfort and decrease anxiety.

Non-nutritive sucking

The use of a pacifier (dummy) is a contentious issue for many parents and children's nurses. Non-nutritive sucking may satisfy a baby's need for contact, making them feel secure and relaxed. It can include sucking on a breast, pacifier, thumb or blanket and can enable the baby to learn about the environment through mouthing objects. Non-nutritive sucking has been effective in some studies in reducing stress in newborns undergoing invasive routine procedures, such as the heel prick test for taking a blood sample (Pinelli and Symington, 2005).

Activity 3.2   *Reflection*

- What are your feelings as a nurse about the use of a dummy?
- If a parent were to come to you and say that their baby was difficult to settle, would you recommend a dummy?
- Are you aware of the evidence base for the use of dummies and the advice given by the Department of Health?

An outline answer is provided at the end of the chapter.

Prayer

Most religions traditionally believe that prayer can cure physical illness and that health can be regained through worship. Baha'is believe in the power of prayer and healing, and the anointing of the sick, and prayer is also very important to Christians. The Church of Jesus Christ of

Latter-day Saints administers spiritual healing to the sick (NHSS, 2006). Buddhist and Hindu traditions believe that illness can be overcome by visiting shrines and praying to gods. A serious diagnosis in a child can present the family with a spiritual crisis, and families often rely on their spiritual or religious beliefs as an important coping strategy.

Spiritual well-being is an important component of holistic health (see 'Holistic care' below). Research has shown that patients have improved clinical outcomes when their care is planned around their faith, religious practices and other personal beliefs (NHSS, 2006). Regardless of its impact on disease, prayer can often help families feel that they are doing everything possible to help their child. Prayer can offer the family a sense of peace and harmony and can reinforce the family's sense of culture and meaning. It is part of the nurse's duty of care to recognise that children have spiritual and religious needs and to meet these needs.

Activity 3.3   *Critical thinking*

It was widely reported that a community nurse was suspended from her post in December 2008 without pay after a complaint about her asking one of her patients if they would like her to 'pray for them'. The nurse, a committed Christian, often handed out home-made prayer cards to her patients and prayed for them. The nurse claimed that her concern was for the patient as a whole, and not just their health.

- Was it unfair of her employers to suspend her without pay?
- What was the nurse doing wrong?
- What part of the NMC *Code* (2008) does this contravene?

Outline answers are provided at the end of the chapter.

Folk medicine

Folk medicine refers to traditional therapies that families use as part of their family or cultural tradition that has been passed down from generation to generation. An example of this is the Hispanic hot–cold belief that illness is derived from an imbalance of the bodily humours (blood, phlegm, black bile and yellow bile). According to this belief system, illness is caused by an imbalance that induces the body to become excessively dry, hot, wet or a combination of these. Therapies are based on the ingestion of plants or other medicines that restore the hot, cold, dry or wet natural balance. Many parents believe that, if they do not wrap their children up warmly, they will 'catch a cold'. Mothers' reliance on home remedies can lead to high rates of non-adherence to prescribed medications. In order to ensure culturally competent practice, you need to be familiar with the folk beliefs and healing practices of the families with which you work.

| Activity 3.4 | Communication |

Luzia is 6 years old and has been admitted for the second time in six months with an acute exacerbation of asthma. Her mother Roberta is Portuguese and has been living in the UK for four years. When you ask her mother about the use of Luzia's regular preventative steroid inhaler, she replies that she only uses the medication when Luzia has acute asthma symptoms, not all the time as prescribed. She confides in you that she believes people in the UK take far too many medicines, and that doctors hide information about medicines from patients. Roberta says she believes that Luzia's asthma is caused by the cold in this country and prefers to prevent the asthma with the use of cod liver oil supplements.

- How do you feel about Roberta's non-compliance with treatment?
- How do you think you should work with Roberta to improve the management of Luzia's care and prevent further readmission to hospital?

Outline answers are provided at the end of the chapter.

Holistic care

Holistic care is about addressing the needs of the child as a whole, which includes body, mind, emotions, spirit and relationships.

Scenario

Judy is a paediatric dermatology nurse specialist and holds nurse-led clinics for patients with atopic eczema. Judy is assessing 10-year-old Arthur, who has eczema for the first time. Judy adopts a holistic approach when assessing Arthur and takes into account the effect of the atopic eczema on Arthur's quality of life. She asks Arthur how the eczema is affecting his sleep and his relationships, and how the eczema makes him feel. Judy is aware that eczema can impact on a child's psychosocial well-being and will take it into consideration when deciding Arthur's treatment plan.

In order to provide holistic care, children's nurses must assess physical, emotional, spiritual, environmental, nutritional and lifestyle needs. Holistic care and assessment must take into consideration the child's and family's values, beliefs, culture and community. The nurse must focus on educating the child and family about lifestyle changes and self-care, and alternative treatment options to drugs and conventional medicines. Parents will often seek out healthcare options that support the child's own natural ability to be healthy. This may be due to concerns about the possible adverse effects of drugs, or simply not wishing to mask a problem with the use of drugs. Healthcare choices for children are mostly made by mothers, and the decisions may be strongly influenced by health professionals such as nurses.

Complementary and alternative medicines

The use of complementary and alternative medicines (CAMs) in the UK is widespread, and although it is difficult to estimate the prevalence rates for use of these therapies in children, greater use is reported in children with chronic illness. Reasons given by parents for using CAMs include:

- to manage the side effects of treatments;
- to cope with the emotional aspects of disease;
- to feel more hopeful;
- to have greater participation in care.

Parents seem to be reluctant to report the use of CAMs to health professionals, and health professionals do not always ask about their use during history taking (Cockayne et al., 2004). As more parents are turning towards the use of CAMs, children's nurses need to be aware of the kinds of therapies parents are using in order to provide basic information on CAM therapies and where to turn for additional information. The children's nurse need not be an expert in every form of CAM therapy, but needs a basic understanding and the ability to seek out the evidence base for CAM practice in order to integrate CAMs into practice.

The term 'complementary' suggests that such care and treatments take place simultaneously with traditional healthcare, whereas 'alternative' implies that such treatments or care take place instead of traditional or conventional medicine. CAMs used in children include homeopathy, chiropractic, music therapy, acupuncture, massage, imagery, touch, dietary and vitamin supplements, herbal products, hypnosis, spiritual healing and prayer. There is limited information about how CAMs affect children. The developmental differences in children mean that they react differently from adults, especially infants and small children. The main concerns around CAMs use in children are safety, efficacy and the potential for interactions with other complementary or pharmaceutical medicines.

CAMs can have side effects, which can differ from side effects in adults. A 'natural' medicine is often mistaken to mean 'safe'. Dietary supplements and herbs can interact with other supplements and medicines. Parents and carers should be encouraged to seek information from rigorous scientific studies when available, rather than relying on **anecdotal evidence**. It is important that, as a registered children's nurse, you have an awareness of the use of CAMs as part of a child's care. You must acknowledge the beliefs that parents have that inform their decision making about the use of CAMs. Interestingly, users of CAMs have been found to be more likely to have a friend or family member in a healthcare profession than non-users of CAMs (Carlton et al., 2009), and CAMs were recommended by them.

Activity 3.5   *Communication*

You are caring for Lloyd, aged 5, who has a diagnosis of acute lymphoblastic leukaemia for which he is undergoing chemotherapy. During conversation, his mother Julie mentions that she is giving Lloyd Chinese herbal medicines and supplements to manage the nausea and vomiting symptoms Lloyd has been experiencing from the chemotherapy. Julie had not

continued opposite . . .

continued . . .

thought to mention this to any of the doctors involved in Lloyd's care, and none of them had asked her if she was using anything herbal. Julie had been informed by the herbalist that it was completely harmless.

- What advice should you give to Julie about this treatment?

An outline answer is provided at the end of the chapter.

A consistent factor of CAM interventions is the aim to comfort, to reduce pain and symptoms and to promote an environment conducive to healing. CAMs can help to ensure that the child or young person feels empowered to manage his or her own responses to the unpleasant or painful situation they find themselves in. There is some evidence that some CAM therapies offer relief of symptoms and may influence healing in children, so there is a place for some therapies in clinical practice. However, there is little scientific evidence available as to whether CAM therapies influence disease processes, increase survival rates, extend life or improve quality of life.

Potential risks and benefits should be determined for therapies that have no evidence, and when CAMs are considered as a substitute or complement to conventional medicine, the child should be referred to an appropriately qualified practitioner to receive such treatment. Children's nurses need to be familiar with a range of CAMs that the parent and child may be using, or may wish to be used in their treatment. The NMC *Code* (2008) states that *You must ensure that the use of complementary or alternative therapies is safe and in the best interest of those in your care.*

Scenario

Judy is a dermatology nurse specialist who holds nurse-led dermatology clinics. She is giving eczema management advice to Kelly, the mother of 2-year-old Eleiyah. Kelly asks for Judy's advice on the use of homeopathy to treat Eleiyah's eczema, as she is considering trying it. Judy informs Kelly that the effectiveness and safety of homeopathy for the management of atopic eczema have not been adequately assessed (NICE, 2007). She advises Kelly that she should continue with the emollients, even if she decides to go ahead with the homeopathy. Judy also asks that Kelly inform her, or any other healthcare professionals providing care to Eleiyah, if she is using homeopathy or any other alternative therapies. This is to ensure that there are no treatment interactions.

The non-pharmacological management of pain and other conditions

The management of pain without the use of medications is called the non-pharmacological management of pain. Each child will experience pain differently, and it is important to discover the best method of pain control for each child. The following methods can be used to manage pain in children and young people.

Psychological strategies

Children are highly imaginative and the unknown and unexpected always seems worse because of this imagination. If the child or young person is adequately prepared and can anticipate what is going to happen to them, their stress levels will be greatly reduced. A children's nurse is able to do this by employing the following strategies.

- Explain all procedures beforehand in detail, using pictures, toys and dolls where available and appropriate. A young child can 'pretend play' the procedure through on a doll or observe a 'demonstration' on a doll.
- Allow the child to meet the doctor/health professional who will perform the procedure beforehand and allow the child to ask questions.
- Allow the child to visit the theatre or treatment room where the procedure will take place.
- An older child or young person can be shown a DVD describing or showing the procedure.

Activity 3.6   *Team working*

During your next ward placement, spend some time observing the play specialist. Ask the play specialist to demonstrate any techniques or toys he or she has for preparing children for clinical procedures.

- Can you think of ways in which you could improve on preparing children psychologically?
- How well do other departments, such as theatre and accident and emergency, prepare children psychologically?

As this activity is an observation of your own practice, there is no outline answer at the end of the chapter.

Distraction therapy

Distraction therapy can be used to help a child cope with a difficult or painful procedure by taking the child's mind off the procedure by concentrating on something else, and has been shown to lessen the reported and observable pain levels in children (Stubenrauch, 2007). Distraction therapy involves getting to know the child's fears and worries about a procedure first (e.g. fear of needles or anaesthetics), then taking time to explain the procedure further, perhaps using play, books, dolls or videos. The type of distraction is then tailored to meet the needs of each child individually and could include reading books, playing games, listening to music, singing, breathing techniques (blowing bubbles, balloons, feathers) and playing with toys (kaleidoscopes, play dough, puppets, dolls). Older children and young people may prefer to just talk about things that interest them or talk through the procedure as it happens. The mind is distracted from the procedure itself by concentrating on the conversation.

Distraction therapy does not work for every child; some children find it very hard to take their minds off a procedure no matter what else is happening around them. In these cases, a different method needs to be used. For some children this may be planning something special they wish to do following the procedure (such as a trip to the park). Just because children can be temporarily distracted from their pain does not mean they do not experience pain or that the pain does not return once the distraction is removed.

Hypnosis and relaxation techniques

With hypnosis a professional such as a psychologist guides the child into an altered state of consciousness that helps the child to focus or narrow their attention in order to reduce discomfort. Relaxation techniques involve guiding the child through relaxation exercises, such as deep breathing and stretching, to reduce discomfort.

Massage

Massage is the physical manipulation of the soft tissues of the body and can be used to produce relaxation. It produces many physical and emotional benefits, including improved circulation of the blood and lymph, and restoration of metabolic balance. The level of contact achieved through massage is an essential component in its effectiveness in reducing pain, anxiety and fear. There is much evidence to support massage as a useful tool for pain management in children when used in combination with other pain management interventions.

Massage can range from giving a scalp or back massage to a hand or foot massage, and can be taught and delegated to family members such as a parent or carer. Giving this task to family members can offer them a feeling of having more control over the situation with their child. The use of baby massage is increasingly popular with healthcare professionals such as health visitors; however, there is insufficient research evidence to support the benefits of baby massage for specific medical conditions such as colic, asthma and dermatitis. There is, however, some evidence that baby massage can benefit the mother–child relationship and reduce postnatal depression.

Aromatherapy

Aromatherapy involves the use of essential oils extracted from aromatic plants as a means of promoting healing, improving well-being and relieving stress. There is no scientific evidence to prove that aromatherapy can cure or prevent disease, but a few studies suggest it can be a useful adjunct for the management of symptoms in some conditions such as cancer. Essential oils are usually massaged into the body, but can also be added to a warm bath or added to a special burner so they are inhaled. Only some of the essential oils are suitable for children; others are not and can be dangerous. Children with epilepsy should not come into contact with stimulating essential oils, for example.

Parents should be advised not to use any aromatherapy on their child without the advice of a qualified aromatherapist. When used correctly, essential oils can be of benefit to some children. Research studies have reported that the essential oil, lavender, may be beneficial in a variety of conditions including insomnia, anxiety, stress and post-operative pain. Essential oils should never be applied neat on to a child's skin but diluted in carrier oil. Massage therapy with the use of essential oils has been tried for the management of childhood atopic eczema; however, one study found a worsening of the eczema after an initial improvement, which suggested a possible allergic contact dermatitis.

Imagery

Imagery is the use of imagination to alter the response to pain, by making it more bearable by substituting a pleasant image in place of pain. It involves guiding the child through a mental image of sights, sounds, smells, tastes and feelings that can help shift attention away from the pain. Pleasant images can be pictured that perhaps are an antidote to the pain; for example, if a child feels a burning pain they can imagine something cool like ice. Children can also be taught to use imagery to imagine that their analgesic drugs are going around their body to the place where the pain is and taking it away. Some children may respond to the concept of a healing ball of light or energy. The child's attention is focused on the healing ball of energy, which travels to the affected painful areas, where it absorbs the pain and takes it away. Imagery is a good method of allowing the child some sense of control over their pain in order to confront and adapt to it (Burns, 2001).

Acupuncture

Acupuncture is a component of traditional Chinese medicine and is based on the theory of a vital energy that circulates throughout the body in 12 channels. When the flow of energy is blocked disease occurs, and when the flow is balanced the patient experiences health. The flow of energy can be affected by stimulating specific points along the energy channels. Most acupuncturists also recommend dietary changes, lifestyle changes, exercise, herbs and other supplements, as well as rest and relationships. Acupuncture has been tried in the management of many childhood conditions, including migraine, allergies, constipation, neurological disabilities, cancer-related conditions, laryngospasm and post-operative vomiting. However, despite many anecdotal reports of success, few scientifically based studies have assessed the effectiveness of acupuncture for children and young people. Much more research is needed to establish an empirical base for the inclusion of acupuncture in standard care.

Chapter summary

This chapter has discussed the role of other health professionals in the management of medicines and alternative treatment options. We have seen the importance of the nurse's role in providing advice on the safe use and availability of over-the-counter medicines for children. Health promotion is an important part of all nursing roles and giving good lifestyle and healthcare advice can help prevent disease and reduce the need for the prescribing and use of medicines within society. In order to provide holistic care, the children's nurse should address the needs of the child as a whole, which includes body, mind, emotions, spirit and relationships. There are alternatives and therapies that are complementary to the use of medicines for the management of many clinical conditions. The children's nurse should allow for individual patient choice, but should ensure that the use of complementary or alternative therapies is safe and in the best interests of the child or young person.

Activities: brief outline answers

Activity 3.2 Use of a dummy (page 75)

The suggestion to use a dummy can stimulate strong feelings from parents and carers, both for and against. Feelings are usually based on social custom, not research evidence, and giving a child a dummy is not known to cause harm. Recent meta-analysis of research by the American Academy of Paediatrics suggests that giving a baby a dummy at the start of any sleep period reduces the risk of cot death. The Department of Health recommends that breastfeeding should be established before a child is given a dummy, which is usually around the age of about 1 month. The DH also recommends that a dummy is gently withdrawn between the ages of 6 and 12 months, as possible adverse effects such as ear infections and dental malocclusions are not unknown. If a dummy falls out once the baby is asleep, it should not be replaced and should never be forced on a baby. It is thought that the degree of protection from cot death is less if a baby who is accustomed to a dummy is not given one (DH, 2009c). If a baby usually has a dummy as part of his or her usual sleep routine, it should be given at every sleep period. Dummies should never be coated with sweet substances such as honey or jam. Two research studies have shown that preterm infants with dummies did not stay in hospital as long as those without dummies.

Activity 3.3 Nurse suspended for offering prayer (page 76)

It would be normal procedure for the nurse to be suspended following such a complaint by a patient, in order to protect the public and allow for further investigation. The nurse had previously been reprimanded for a similar incident and it is likely her colleagues were concerned about her conduct. The nurse had a strong faith and, although the nurse meant well, she was in a position of trust and could be considered to be forcing her faith on her patients. The NMC *Code* (2008) states that *You must not use your professional status to promote causes that are not related to health.* You could argue, however, that the nurse believed in holistic care, and prayer is a part of this. But you do not know your patients' beliefs and preferences, and some may be offended. The NMC *Code* (2008) also states that *You must demonstrate a personal and professional commitment to equality and diversity.*

You must never force your faith on a patient; however, it is appropriate to respond impartially if patients themselves bring up the subject of religion.

Activity 3.4 Lack of adherence to treatment (page 77)

Did you feel that Roberta's failure to 'comply' with treatment was somehow being irrational, irresponsible, deviant or simply ignorant? If we apply a parent-focused approach to care, we can understand that Roberta's behaviour, while 'non-compliant' from our perspective, is logically consistent with her own belief system and the way she makes sense of the asthma. It is now preferable to talk about 'adherence' to treatment rather than 'compliance'.

Often a family's belief about the nature, cause and preventative management of illness differs from evidence-based medical practice. Parents will often maintain their folk beliefs and practices without ever discussing them or confirming their validity with health professionals. Roberta's reluctance to use the prescribed medication for the prevention of asthma is based on a mistrust of standard medical practice, which is in conflict with her traditional and cultural beliefs about illness in general. Roberta does not see herself as being non-compliant or failing to provide adequate care. However, by our standards and beliefs based on research evidence, the care Roberta is offering Luzia is inadequate and not in the best interests of the child.

It is important that children's nurses acknowledge the folk beliefs of parents and the home remedies they use in order to find ways to bring together differences. Just holding the view that we can educate parents about Western standards and our beliefs is not enough. We need to explore in depth the parent's belief about the causes and treatments of asthma. It is important that we recognise that parents' beliefs about illness and treatment extend further than medical and biological boundaries to their social and cultural backgrounds. We must attempt to reconcile contradictory practices by using a negotiated approach to 'concordance'.

Activity 3.5 Parent administering Chinese herbal medicine (pages 78–9)

Julie administering a Chinese herbal medicine to Lloyd without informing the doctors is potentially very dangerous. Little is known about the effect of herbal remedies or nutritional supplements in combination with chemotherapy. Most supplements available over the counter are not standardised and some products have been known to contain misidentified plants. Although a qualified medical herbalist would not prescribe any remedies that interact with orthodox medication, the herbal medicine Julie is administering to Lloyd could interfere with the therapeutic action of the chemotherapy or increase the toxicity of the chemotherapy, leading to harm. You should discuss the implications of this with Julie and request her permission to discuss this with the medical staff in order to ensure that any treatments are safe.

Further reading

Department of Health (DH) (2008) *The Child Health Promotion Programme: Pregnancy and the first five years of life*. London: Department of Health.

This sets out the standard for delivery of the Child Health Promotion Programme, and concentrates on the first few years of life.

Department of Health (DH) (2009) *Birth to Five*. London: Department of Health.

This is a key Department of Health publication that is free to all parents in England and is available on the department's website at **www.dh.gov.uk**. You will find in this book the information advice for parents on the management of common childhood illnesses and other useful health promotion information and advice.

Mantle, F (2004) *Complementary and Alternative Medicine for Child and Adolescent Care*. London: Butterworth-Heinemann.

This book is a useful complementary and alternative medicine text for nurses working with children and young people. The book covers broad aspects of professional and safety issues and an overview of CAM therapies.

National Health Service Scotland (NHSS) (2009) *Spiritual Care Matters: An introductory resource for all NHS Scotland staff*. Edinburgh: NHS Education for Scotland.

Useful websites

http://nccam.nih.gov

The website of the US National Center for Complementary and Alternative Medicine.

www.education.gov.uk

This Department of Education website includes information on Sure Start Children's Centres.

www.eatwell.gov.uk

This website gives advice on eating more healthily and how to eat less saturated fat. The eatwell plate helps healthy eating easier to understand.

www.fsid.org.uk

The Foundation for the Study of Infant Death promotes safe baby care advice.

www.healthystart.nhs.uk

The Healthy Start site offers advice to families receiving certain benefits on how to get free milk, vitamins, fruit and vegetables.

www.mhra.gov.uk/NewsCentre/CON028268

This web page from the Medicines and Healthcare products Regulatory Agency provides guidance and advice on the safe use of medicines and medical devices. You will find the new advice on children's over-the-counter cough and cold medicines.

www.nhs.uk/change4life/Pages/change-for-life.aspx

Change4Life is a nationwide campaign designed to help people make changes to their lifestyle in order to stay healthy and live longer.

www.nhs.uk/Livewell

The Live Well website contains hundreds of articles on many topics around staying healthy.

www.schoolfoodtrust.org.uk

The School Food Trust aims to transform school food and food skills and promote the education and health of children and young people.

Chapter 4
Knowledge of children's medicines and their actions

NMC Standards for Pre-registration Nursing Education

This chapter will address the following competencies:

Domain 3: Nursing practice and decision-making

Field standard for competence:

Children's nurses must be able to care safely and effectively for children and young people in all settings, and recognise their responsibility for safeguarding them. They must be able to deliver care to meet essential and complex physical and mental health needs informed by deep understanding of biological, psychological and social factors throughout infancy, childhood and adolescence.

Competencies:

2. All nurses must possess a broad knowledge of the structure and functions of the human body, and other relevant knowledge from the life, behavioural and social sciences as applied to health, ill health, disability, ageing and death. They must have an in-depth knowledge of common physical and mental health problems and treatments in their own field of practice, including co-morbidity and physiological and psychological vulnerability.

3. All nurses must carry out comprehensive, systematic nursing assessments that take account of relevant physical, social, cultural, psychological, spiritual, genetic and environmental factors, in partnership with service users and others through interaction, observation and measurement.

3.1 **Children's nurses** must carry out comprehensive nursing assessments of children and young people, recognising the particular vulnerability of infants and young children to rapid physiological deterioration.

4. All nurses must ascertain and respond to the physical, social and psychological needs of people, groups and communities. They must then plan, deliver and evaluate safe, competent, person-centred care in partnership with them, paying special attention to changing health needs during different life stages, including progressive illness and death, loss and bereavement.

Chapter aims

By the end of this chapter, you should be able to:

- understand how drugs are absorbed, metabolised and excreted;
- appreciate the anatomical and physiological differences in children that need to be considered in drug regimes;
- understand how drugs exert their effects on the body;
- describe basic drug interactions.

Case study

The bodies of babies and children do not deal with drugs in the same way as those of adults. In the past, a lack of knowledge of these developmental differences has led to unexpected complications of drug therapy in children. For example, some newborn children died from side effects of the antibiotic chloramphenicol (Lischner et al., 1961). It was not known that premature babies and neonates lacked the liver enzymes necessary to metabolise the drug, leading to the accumulation of toxic chloramphenicol metabolites. Symptoms would include vomiting, cyanosis, hypotension and an ashen grey colour of skin. It became known as 'grey baby syndrome'. If the antibiotic was not stopped, the infant would develop hypothermia and cardiovascular collapse, and would often die. For this reason chloramphenicol is not usually administered to neonates or premature babies.

Introduction

'Children are not small adults' is a saying frequently used to put across the complexities of developmental differences that alter the nature of drug actions in infants, children and young people. Children's body systems are less developed, their gastrointestinal transit time varies, and their body composition changes with development. It is important that the developmental stage of a child is taken into consideration when a nurse is administering medications, in order to ensure that safe therapeutic drug regimes are adhered to.

This chapter will explain the differences in the absorption, distribution, metabolism and excretion of medications during infancy and childhood, and the way this affects how we as nurses administer medicines to children.

Pharmacokinetics

Pharmacokinetics is the term used to describe how the body handles a drug over a period of time, including how it absorbs, distributes, metabolises and excretes the drug (from the Greek *pharma* = drug, *kineo* = move). In other words, it describes what the body does to the drug. In order for a drug to be effective, it must be available at the site of action in the correct concentration.

Absorption

Absorption is the process by which a drug moves from the site of entry into the body, such as the gastrointestinal tract or a muscle, into the circulatory or lymphatic system. The developmental stage of the child presents a distinctive range of factors that will affect the efficiency and rate of drug absorption. The child's disease state or illness may also affect drug absorption.

The rate of absorption is influenced by:

- the dosage form;
- the chemical properties of the drug;
- the circulation at the site of absorption;
- the surface area that the drug is exposed to;
- the contact time of the drug with the absorption site;
- drug–drug and food–drug interactions;
- the route of administration.

Dosage form

The dosage form refers to the drug's physical state, which can be either liquid or solid. Many medicines for children come in liquid form, which can be **suspensions**, **elixirs**, **aqueous solutions** or oil based. Solid drug formulations include plain tablets, **soluble**, **sustained release** and **modified release** tablets, **enteric coated** tablets, and **capsules**. Other solid drug formulations are **suppositories**, **creams**, **ointments** and **emollients**. Drugs must be in solution to be absorbed, so solid forms must be able to disintegrate. Drugs in elixir or syrup formulation are absorbed faster than tablets or capsules. Medicines administered intravenously have the most rapid onset of action. In general, medicines administered in high doses are generally absorbed more quickly than those given in low concentrations.

Chemical properties

The chemical property of a drug is its chemical formation, which will affect how it behaves in the body. Factors that will influence the drug's behaviour and how it moves across tissues in the body are:

* the drug's fat solubility or water solubility;
* the size and shape of the molecules;
* the drug acidity/alkalinity (**pH**);
* **ionisation**;
* salt composition.

A drug must cross several semi-permeable cell membranes in order to reach the circulation (unless it is given intravenously). Cell membranes are biological barriers that selectively inhibit the passage of drug molecules. Cell membranes are composed mainly of double layers of fat cells (mostly cholesterol-based), which determine the kind of substances they will let pass through.

Drugs may cross cell membranes by:

* passive diffusion;
* facilitated passive diffusion;
* active transport;
* pinocytosis.

Passive diffusion

Passive diffusion is the movement of material across a cell membrane from an area of high concentration to an area of low concentration. The rate of diffusion is directly proportional to the diffusion gradient, which is the difference in concentration either side of the cell membrane. Diffusion will continue across the cell membrane until this gradient has been eliminated. Since diffusion moves materials from an area of high concentration to an area of low concentration, it is described as moving solutes 'down the concentration gradient'. Other factors such as the size of the molecule, its lipid solubility, degree of ionisation and area of absorption will also influence the process. Small molecules tend to penetrate cell membranes more rapidly than larger molecules, and because the cell membrane is lipoid, lipid-soluble drugs diffuse more rapidly. Most drugs are weak acids or bases that exist in either an ionised or un-ionised form when dissolved in water. Un-ionised forms are usually lipid-soluble and diffuse readily across cell membranes. Ionised forms have low lipid solubility, but high water solubility, and so cannot penetrate cell membranes easily (see Figure 4.1).

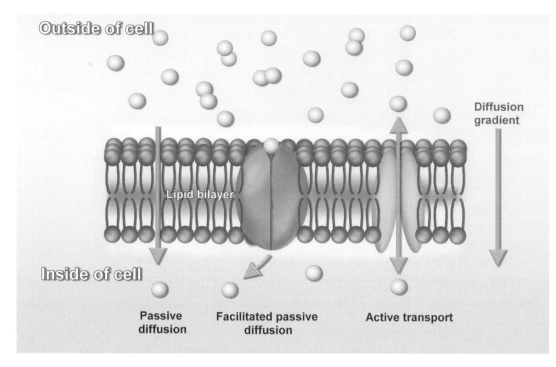

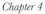

Figure 4.1: Passive diffusion

Facilitated passive diffusion

Facilitated passive diffusion is when proteins are used to help move molecules more quickly. Glucose is a good example, and as most cells use glucose for energy, this mechanism is important. Since the cell membrane will not allow glucose to cross by diffusion, help is needed. The cell membrane carrier molecule combines with the glucose molecule in order to diffuse it rapidly across the cell membrane and release it into the cell. The glucose is moving down a concentration gradient from a higher to lower concentration and does not require energy (see Figure 4.1).

Active transport

Active transport requires energy expenditure and can occur against a concentration gradient. The proteins embedded in the cell's lipid bilayer do much of the work in active transport. The proteins are positioned to cross the membrane so that one part is on the inside of the cell and one part is on the outside. The proteins are able to move molecules and ions in and out of the cell. Active transport seems to be limited to drugs that have a similar appearance to substances naturally produced in the body, such as vitamins, sugars and amino acids, and are usually absorbed from specific sites in the small intestine (see Figure 4.1).

Pinocytosis

Pinocytosis is the engulfing of particles or fluid by the cell. Energy expenditure is required for pinocytosis, which probably plays a small role in drug transport. The cell membrane **invaginates** in order to enclose the particle or fluid, and then unites again forming a **vesicle** that detaches and moves to the interior of the cell (see Figure 4.2).

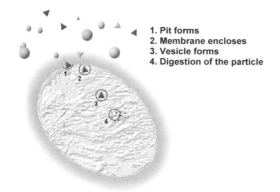

1. Pit forms
2. Membrane encloses
3. Vesicle forms
4. Digestion of the particle

Figure 4.2: Pinocytosis

The circulation at the site of absorption

The absorption and distribution of a drug depends on the patient's blood circulation, and is better in areas that are well **perfused** than in areas with sluggish circulation. For example, in cardiac arrest, an intravenously administered drug will be unable to reach its target organ unless an effective circulation is restored.

The surface area that the drug is exposed to

Absorption of a drug into the systemic circulation is favourable if adequate concentration of the drug is exposed to a large surface area with a good blood supply. It is helpful if the surface area happens to be the required site of the drug's action, for example topical steroids in the treatment of skin disorders and inhaled bronchodilators in the management of asthma.

The contact time with the drug

The longer the contact time with the site of absorption, the higher the concentration of drug absorbed. The differences in gastric emptying time and gut motility in infants and children as opposed to those of adults, and also some clinical conditions, are important factors to consider in oral medicines administration.

Drug–drug and food–drug interactions

Absorption can be influenced by the presence of food or other drugs in the stomach. The presence of food in the stomach may decrease or increase the rate and extent of drug absorption, and drugs may influence nutrient absorption. For example:

*   the antibiotics ciprofloxacin and tetracycline form an insoluble complex with calcium in dairy products, supplements or antacids, decreasing drug absorption;
*   absorption of the antibiotic cefuroxime can be enhanced by the presence of food in the stomach;
*   food ingested at the same time as the beta-blocker propranolol reduces the first pass metabolism in the liver, resulting in higher serum drug levels;
*   the anticonvulsants phenobarbital and phenytoin increase the metabolism of folic acid and vitamins D and K, with the risk of deficiencies.

For these reasons you must always check for interactions in the BNFC and follow the instructions for administration given by the pharmacist. You should advise parents of the importance of following any instructions for when to adminster medicines. 'With' or 'after food' means take the medicine at the same time as a meal or directly following to avoid the medicine irritating the stomach. 'Before food' means on an empty stomach, which should be at least an hour before a meal, so that the acids released during the meal do not destroy the medicine.

Now try the following activity, which is to enable you to reflect on how safely and effectively you administer a commonly prescribed drug that works at the site of application.

Activity 4.1   *Reflection*

- When administering topical anaesthetics to children, such as EMLA cream, what is the recommended dosage advice for a child aged 1–3 months?
- What is the difference between the dose for a child of 1–3 months and for a child aged 1–18 years? What do you think the reasons for this are?

Outline answers are provided at the end of the chapter.

Route of administration

The route of administration that is chosen (oral, intravenous, etc.) may have a profound effect upon the speed and efficacy with which the medicine acts. The most appropriate route of administration must be chosen according to the intended therapeutic purpose of the medicine and the licensing and formulations (see Chapter 6). The route of administration will determine the drug dosage, as the route chosen will influence the rate and extent of drug absorption, a concept known as bioavailability.

Bioavailability

Bioavailability is defined as the fraction of the administered drug dose that reaches the systemic circulation. For all intravenous administration the bioavailability is 100 per cent. Other routes of administration vary from 0 to 100 per cent. For example, the bioavailability of paracetamol tablets is 100 per cent compared to 93 per cent for paracetamol suppositories. Hence, there is very little therapeutic advantage in using the intravenous form, and oral formulations should be used whenever possible.

Factors influencing bioavailability include the drug's chemical properties, drug formulation, route of administration, body surface area, blood flow and contact time. A drug that is not very soluble through cell membranes will have low bioavailability. The degree of first pass metabolism (see below) will also influence bioavailability. The bioavailability of morphine oral solution is about 24 per cent, controlled release oral tablet 22.5 per cent and buccal tablet 19 per cent. Intravenous morphine has a bioavailability of 100 per cent; hence, much smaller doses need to be given intravenously compared to enterally.

The next activity is to enable you to reflect on the differences between oral and intravenous dosages in children.

Activity 4.2   *Decision making*

Lydia is 12 years old and weighs 39kg and has been prescribed paracetamol 500mg every 4–6 hours for pain following dental extractions. However, she is unable to tolerate the medicine orally as she is vomiting. The prescribing doctor has written the dose up to be given by rectum.

- What would the correct rectal dose for Lydia be?

Lydia refuses the suppository; however, she has a patent cannula in situ following surgery.

- Would this be an appropriate route for the paracetamol and, if so, what is the correct dose?

Outline answers are provided at the end of the chapter.

First pass metabolism

First pass metabolism refers to the first pass through the liver of substances absorbed into the hepatic portal vein after digestion. It greatly reduces the concentration of a drug before it reaches the systemic circulation. After a medicine is taken orally, it is absorbed by the gut and enters the hepatic portal system, where it is carried to the liver by the portal vein before it reaches the rest of the body. Some drugs are metabolised by the liver to such an extent that only a small amount of the active drug emerges from the liver and enters the systemic circulation. Hence, the first pass through the liver greatly reduces the bioavailability of some drugs. Morphine is subject to extensive first pass metabolism. Alternative routes of administration such as intravenous, intramuscular, inhalation, suppository and sublingual avoid the first pass effect and allow the drug to be absorbed directly into the systemic circulation.

The following activity will help you to reflect on the differences in oral medicine doses compared to other routes due to first pass metabolism in the liver.

Activity 4.3   *Critical thinking*

Michael is 13 years old, weighs 50kg and has been prescribed morphine for his pain.

- What would be the correct dosage range of morphine for Michael orally, intravenously and intramuscularly?
- Can you explain the reason for this variation in dose?

Outline answers are provided at the end of the chapter.

Anatomical and physiological differences between neonates, children and young people

Although children may often receive the same medicines via similar routes as adults do, the child's growth, difference in fluid distribution, immaturity of body systems and physiological development can exaggerate or diminish the effectiveness of some drug regimes. Medicine dosages consequently vary greatly in children and need to be calculated individually, usually by weight in kilograms or body surface area (BSA; see also 'Weight and body surface area' on pages 12–13).

The key points of pharmacokinetics for infants and children are as follows.

- Babies and small children are unable to tell us if they are experiencing side effects from medicines.
- The lack of clinical trials in children means that there is a poor evidence base for safer prescribing.
- There is a greater likelihood of side effects in preterm babies and neonates.
- Doses need to be calculated individually, either by weight in kilograms or by body surface area.
- Fat to water ratios are different in children.
- Limited protein binding (see page 100) gives a greater amount of free drug in circulation.
- Immature enzyme function (0–1 year) means slower metabolism of many drugs.
- Excretion by the kidneys is less developed in infants, leading to slower elimination of renally cleared drugs and their metabolites.

Oral absorption

The oral route is the most frequent and suitable method of administering medicines to children. The absorption of oral drugs involves transport across epithelial cell membranes into the gastrointestinal tract. To be absorbed orally, a drug must undergo exposure to low pH and numerous degrading enzymes. Some drugs such as insulin are particularly susceptible to degradation and are therefore not used orally. Factors influencing absorption include the pH along the gastrointestinal tract, the surface area of the **lumen**, blood perfusion and presence of bile or mucus, and the type of epithelial membranes.

Buccal and sublingual absorption

The oral mucosa has a rich blood supply and a thin membrane that favours absorption; however, most medicines do not remain in contact with the oral mucosa long enough to be absorbed. Some medicines are formulated for buccal administration (placed between the gums and the cheek) or sublingual administration (under the tongue), where they are retained longer, thus enhancing absorption. Opioids are absorbed rapidly by this route, and buccal midazolam administration offers an effective treatment for prolonged seizures in children.

Swallowing

Choking and the aspiration of medicines into the airway is a risk in infants and young children due to the small diameter of the oesophagus and the anatomy of the pharynx. It is recommended that tablets or capsules are not offered to children under 5 years. Most tablets and capsules are designed for adults and are too difficult for children to swallow safely. Small children can also choke on chewable tablets. Crushing tablets and opening capsules can alter the intended absorption process and the drug action, so seek advice from a pharmacist before doing this. Wherever possible, liquid formulations should be prescribed for younger children and those unable to swallow tablets safely.

Gastric pH

The newborn term infant tends to have more neutral gastric juice at birth (pH 6–8) due to the presence of amniotic fluid in the stomach that has been swallowed in the uterus. This falls to more acidic values within the first 48 hours. The immaturity of the gastric mucosal cells in secreting hydrochloric acid influences the gastric pH. Adult pH values are reached by the age of 3 months. In premature infants gastric pH may remain high due to immature gastric acid secretion and may lead to less degradation of certain drugs such as penicillin, leading to increased absorption. Absorption of drugs that are pH dependent, such as phenobarbital, paracetamol and riboflavin (vitamin B2), will be delayed. The development of the gastric mucosa usually reaches adult levels of gastric acid production by about 3–5 years of age.

Gastric emptying time

Gastric emptying time is an important factor in the absorption of drugs as most oral drugs are absorbed in the jejunum. Most drugs administered orally to young children are given in liquid form, which is absorbed more quickly than the solid form. Prolonged drug exposure in the stomach of preterm infants who have delayed gastric emptying time may alter the rate and extent of absorption of the drug. Some oral medicines are therefore slower to reach their peak concentrations in neonates. Delayed absorption is not often of clinical importance unless high peak plasma concentrations are required quickly, for example when administering analgesia. Gastrointestinal transit times are generally prolonged in infants under 6 months, leading to increased degradation of some drugs. Older infants are more likely to have intestinal hurry, that is, shortened gastrointestinal transit times, leading to reduced amounts of drug being absorbed.

Gastrointestinal drug absorption may also be affected during illnesses such as gastroenteritis and related diarrhoea. The structural and functional changes to the intestinal mucosa of infants with prolonged diarrhoea can facilitate the absorption of some drugs (e.g. gentamicin, which is not usually absorbed from the gut) and impair the absorption of others. Children with malabsorption syndromes, such as coeliac disease and cystic fibrosis, may experience a reduction in absorption of digoxin and antibiotics, and delayed prednisolone absorption occurs in inflammatory bowel disease. Infants with congenital heart disease may have prolonged gastric emptying times, leading to diminished absorption ability.

Intravenous absorption

Intravenous injection is the preferred route of medicines administration when rapid onsets of action or a constant therapeutic drug concentration is required. Administering medicines intravenously will avoid the first pass metabolism that occurs with oral administration, so may be a route of choice, for example, with morphine, which undergoes extensive first pass metabolism if given orally. This may also be the route of choice when a child is vomiting or nil by mouth for some reason. The intravenous route in infants and children offers the fastest onset of drug action, but is also the most dangerous. Once injected the medication cannot be retrieved and will take effect almost immediately. Care must be taken that equipment is not contaminated with pathogens, which would have direct access to the systemic circulation and could lead to septicaemia.

Intramuscular absorption

The intramuscular route is one of the least preferred methods of medicines administration in children as it is painful and children are reluctant to cooperate. Absorption is erratic and dependent upon muscle blood flow, which can be diminished due to age and clinical condition. The small muscle mass in neonates, infants and young children limits the volume of medicine that can be administered at any site.

Intraosseus absorption

Intraosseus infusions involve injections of medications or fluids directly into the bone marrow when the intravenous route cannot be established quickly, usually in paediatric emergencies. Intraosseus infusions have roughly the same absorption rates as intravenous infusions, and allow for fluid resuscitation and high-volume drugs to be administered quickly.

Topical absorption

A number of medicines can be administered to children topically. Medicines applied topically in order to have a systemic effect (contraceptive patch or nicotine patch) diffuse through the epidermis of the skin to reach the capillary network and systemic circulation. Medicines applied topically to have a local effect diffuse into the area immediately below the administration site, such as the subcutaneous tissue (eczema treatment) or muscle (local anaesthetics). Absorption is dependent on a variety of factors including:

- site of application;
- thickness of the **stratum corneum** and skin integrity;
- skin hydration status (increased hydration enhances absorption);
- pH of the drug;
- lipid solubility and molecule size;
- skin perfusion, which may be altered by the disease state (shock), temperature and drug action.

Major considerations when administering topical medications to children are toxic effects and limiting the uptake of the drug (AAP, 1997). Infants and children have a relatively rich blood supply combined with well-hydrated, thinner skin, which can lead to increased absorption of topical applications. This can be considered advantageous in some instances, but can be a disadvantage, leading to systemic toxicity. Absorption will be high in infants due to their skin surface area being high in relation to body weight. Greater absorption occurs where skin is inflamed or broken. Areas where skin is thinner, such as the face, eyelids and genital area, and flexural sites such as the axillae and groin, also have greater absorption. Absorption is increased also by **occlusion**, for example applying the occlusive dressing over EMLA cream.

Skin washes such as chlorhexidine and povidine-iodine should be used with caution in neonates due to their thin skin and large body surface area, which would allow toxic levels to develop from systemic absorption. Alcohol preparations should be avoided in neonates because they can dehydrate the skin and can cause necrosis (BMA et al., 2010). Topical corticosteroids should be used with care in neonates and infants as absorption through the skin can, if over-administered, cause adrenal suppression and even **Cushing's syndrome**.

Fatalities have occurred in children from topical medication administration, often due to accidental absorption through mucous membranes, such as the mouth from sucking and mucous membranes of the eye through rubbing. Absorption of EMLA cream through a mucous membrane, for example if a child sucks on the cream or rubs it into the eye, may cause toxic effects (AAP, 1997).

Transdermal hyoscine patches are effective for the prevention of motion sickness in children over 10 years. The patch should be applied behind the ear, which should prevent the child from rubbing the patch in the eye, which has been known to cause mydriasis (prolonged dilatation of the pupil) (AAP, 1997).

Rectal absorption

Rectal administration provides the rapid absorption of many drugs and may be an appropriate alternative to other routes for the management and treatment of nausea and vomiting, seizures, pain and fever. Absorption occurs through the rectal mucosa in order to obtain systemic effects of a medicine. The rectal route is relatively painless and less threatening than some other routes; however, it may not be socially or culturally acceptable for some children. Rectal administration of medicines should be avoided in children who are immunosuppressed, as even minimal trauma can lead to abscess formation.

The uptake of rectally administered medicines can be erratic and variability from child to child exists. Drug absorption can be prolonged or delayed and you should be aware of this factor and avoid the temptation of giving multiple doses when effects are delayed. The rate of rectal transmucosal absorption is affected by:

- the physical properties of the suppository and the time it takes to dissolve;
- the volume of the medicine;
- the concentration of the medicine;
- the presence of stool in the rectum;
- the pH of the rectal contents;
- the retention of the administered medicine;
- the venous drainage of the rectum.

The clinical implications of rectal venous drainage for absorption and metabolism are not clear for most drugs. It is thought that medicines administered high in the rectum will enter the superior rectal veins and are usually carried directly to the liver to undergo first pass metabolism. Drugs administered low in the rectum enter the inferior and middle rectal veins and enter the systemic circulation before passing through the liver; this can affect the bioavailability of drugs that have a high hepatic extraction ratio.

The pH range of most children's rectums favours the absorption of barbiturates, such as diazepam and midazolam, and is convenient for the treatment of status epilepticus.

The key points of rectal absorption are:

- the onset of effect takes minutes;
- the duration of effect lasts for hours;
- drug absorption varies considerably from child to child;
- the child may expel some of the drug, which is impossible to measure;
- dosages are limited by the fixed sizes of suppositories.

Breastfeeding

Almost all drugs a mother takes orally will cross into breast milk, but mostly in such small quantities that they will not affect the infant. There are few contraindications for breastfeeding when it is necessary for a mother to take medications. However, breastfeeding mothers should only take medication that is absolutely necessary. Preterm and jaundiced infants are at a slightly higher risk of toxicity if the drug enters the mother's milk in significant quantities.

For example, sulphonamides (a broad spectrum antibiotic) should not be administered in late pregnancy or to breastfeeding mothers, because of the risk of jaundice and haemolytic anaemia due to the **bilirubin** in the baby's blood being displaced by the sulphonamide. **Kernicterus** can occur when excess bilirubin penetrates the blood–brain barrier, leading to brain damage, vision and hearing problems and cerebral palsy.

The next activity is to enable you to reflect and feel confident in giving advice to a breastfeeding mother who herself is taking medication.

Activity 4.4   *Communication*

Joel is 5 days old and he is being exclusively breastfed. His mother has been prescribed warfarin as she developed a deep vein thrombosis following the surgery for Joel's Caesarean birth. His mother knows it is essential that she continues on the warfarin due to being at risk of a pulmonary embolism, and is very concerned that the warfarin will pass through her breast milk and cause Joel side effects such as bleeding.

- What advice would you give Joel's mother?

An outline answer is provided at the end of the chapter.

Distribution

Distribution involves the transport of drugs around the body, and the simplest factor determining how much drug is distributed is the amount of blood flow to the body tissues. Organs such as the liver, heart, kidneys and brain receive the most blood supply, so it is easy to deliver high concentrations of drugs to these organs. In contrast, the skin, bone and fat tissues receive less blood flow, so it is more difficult to deliver high concentrations of drugs. Again, the physical property of the drug will have an effect on how it moves throughout the body after it has been administered. The lipid solubility of a drug is an important factor as this will determine how it is absorbed, circulates in the blood, crosses cell membranes and is deposited in body tissue. Drugs that are lipid soluble are not restricted by the barriers that would prevent the distribution of water-soluble drugs and are therefore more completely distributed throughout the body tissues. Tissues such as fat, bone marrow, teeth and eyes are highly affinitive to some medications and have the ability to accumulate and store drugs after absorption. Barbiturates such as thiopental, which is used in general anaesthesia, and diazepam, a benzodiazepine, are highly attractive to adipose tissue, along with the fat-soluble vitamins. The antibiotic tetracycline binds with calcium salts and can accumulate in the bones and teeth. When drugs are stored in body tissue they can remain in the body for months to be slowly released back into the circulation.

The following activity is to enable you to reflect on drugs that are distributed differently in children.

Activity 4.5 — *Critical thinking*

Tamara is 10 years old and has been prescribed the antibiotic tetracycline for a diagnosis of pneumonia by her GP.

* Why is this drug inappropriate for her?

An outline answer is provided at the end of the chapter.

Body composition

Differences in the ratio of lean body weight to fat can alter drug distribution, leading to changes in the pharmacological response. Infants and younger children have a greater percentage of body water and extracellular fluid and less body fat. This means the percentage of body water and fats is different in infants and younger children, compared to older children and adults. This can lead to a larger volume of distribution of water-soluble drugs in infants and younger children due to extended water volumes. However, reduced body fat may lead to a decrease in the retention of fat-soluble drugs.

As a child gets older:

* total body water and extracellular fluid reduces;
* total fat increases.

Neonates:

* need higher doses of water-soluble drugs per kilogram of body weight;
* need lower doses of fat-soluble drugs per kilogram of body weight.

Table 4.1 gives a rough estimate of the body fat/water composition at different ages throughout the lifespan. You can see that children contain much higher percentages of body water, and less

	Percentage body water	**Percentage body fat**
Preterm infant	80	6
Newborn infant	73–77	13
Toddler 1 year	60	22
10-year-old child	65	14
Adult male	60 (47 in obese man)	8–17 (35 in obese man)
Adult female	52	14–21

Table 4.2: Water and fat composition of the body

body fat. Also, women in general contain more body fat than men. Individuals who are more muscular and athletic, and are leaner, will have less body fat. (The rest of the body content would be made up of varying amounts of proteins and minerals.)

The next activity is to enable you to reflect on the prescribing of medicines in relation to body fat/water composition.

Activity 4.6   *Critical thinking*

Bertie is 7 years old and appears to be grossly obese. He weighs 35kg and his height is 122cm.

• How should drug dosages for Bertie be calculated?

An outline answer is provided at the end of the chapter.

Plasma protein binding

Another factor that can affect the distribution of drugs is the binding capacity of plasma proteins. Drugs that have entered the systemic circulation are delivered to the tissues via the blood. The plasma proteins within the blood are capable of forming bonds with drugs (drug–protein complexes) that are reversible and non-selective. Acidic drugs will tend to bind to albumin and bases will bind to globulins, lipoproteins and glycoproteins. Drug–protein complexes are too large to cross capillary membranes. Drugs bound to proteins are categorised as inactive, as only the free unbound drug will have a pharmacological effect. Drugs bound to proteins circulate in the plasma until they are released or displaced from the drug–protein complex. A large number of drugs are strongly bound to plasma proteins in such a way that there is very little free drug or chemical in the circulation. Only the free drug can be excreted by the kidney, be taken up by the liver or enter the central nervous system. Extensive protein binding will delay the elimination of a drug and will also limit the amount of drug that is free to exert its effects.

Serum albumin and total plasma protein concentrations are reduced during infancy and only come close to adult levels by about 1 year of age. Reduced plasma protein binding of drugs in infants results in an increase of free drug and the possibility of drug toxicity. Conditions that cause a reduction in serum albumin and plasma proteins, such as malnutrition and cystic fibrosis, will cause alterations in the protein binding of drugs, leading to increased amounts of free drug. Children with malignancies or burns, or who have undergone trauma or surgery, may have increased plasma protein, which enhances the binding of basic drugs.

Blood–brain barrier and foetal placental barrier

The brain and the placenta have distinctive anatomical barriers that prevent many drugs from passing through. Medicines used for anxiety, sedation and epilepsy will readily pass through the blood–brain barrier to exert their effects on the central nervous system. However, most anti-cancer drugs do not easily pass this barrier, making brain cancers difficult to treat. The foetal placental barrier prevents potentially harmful substances from passing from the mother's blood to the foetus. However, substances such as caffeine, alcohol, cocaine and some prescription medications easily cross the placental barrier and can lead to birth defects.

Metabolism

Metabolism is the process of chemically converting a drug to a form that is usually more easily removed from the body. Metabolism is also called biotransformation and involves complex biochemical pathways and reactions that alter drugs. The primary site of drug metabolism is the liver, but the kidney, intestinal tract, skin and lungs may also play a part. When drugs pass through the liver they undergo phase 1 chemical reactions, such as hydrolysis, hydroxylation, oxidation and reduction. In phase 2, side chains known as conjugates are added to make the drug more water soluble and more easily excreted by the kidneys.

Liver enzyme activity

Metabolism in the liver is achieved by a complex system of enzymes called the **hepatic microsomal enzyme system**, commonly known as the P-450 system (named after a key component of the system, cytochrome P-450). The purpose of the P-450 system is to inactivate drugs and accelerate their excretion. Some drugs can be chemically altered by this system to be made more active by metabolism, for example codeine is chemically transformed to morphine, which is more active at relieving pain. Other drugs known as **prodrugs** are administered in an inactive form and need to be metabolised by the body before they become active and have any pharmacological effect. The antiviral drug acyclovir is an example of a prodrug; it is administered in an inactive (or less active) form and is metabolised into a more active drug after administration.

Some drugs have the ability to increase enzyme activity in the liver. For example, phenobarbital causes the liver to produce more microsomal enzymes, thereby increasing the rate of its own metabolism and the need for dosing to be adjusted.

Factors influencing metabolism

Any child with decreased liver function, such as in liver disease or genetic disorders in which children lack specific enzymes (e.g. glucose-6-phosphate dehydrogenase), will need their drug doses to be adjusted accordingly. Liver enzyme activity is very much dependent on a person's age and is generally reduced in infants and children. Oxidising enzyme activity is greatly reduced. The newborn's reduced enzyme activity results in the prolonged elimination of drugs such as diazepam and phenytoin. The pathway responsible for the metabolism of paracetamol, caffeine and toxic substances such as cigarette smoke is about one-third of adult activity in the infant, and only reaches adult levels at about 10 years of age.

Excretion

Excretion is the process by which substances, including drugs, are removed from the body. The rate of excretion will affect the concentration of drugs in the bloodstream and body tissues. The concentration of drugs in the bloodstream will determine their duration of action. Drugs are removed from the body by numerous organs and tissues, including the kidney (in the urine) and the liver (in the bile), and are excreted in saliva, sweat, tears and the breath. For example, alcohol is partly excreted in the breath, which enables the police to test drivers with breath alcohol testing devices. The majority of drugs are excreted in bile and urine. Kidney glomerular filtration rate and tubular secretion and reabsorption will all have an impact on the excretion of drugs or their water-soluble metabolites. The development of the nephron in the foetus continues up to 36 weeks gestational age. The overall functional capacity of the kidney increases with age up to early adulthood. The filtration of drugs through the glomerulus is dependent on:

- the functional capacity of the glomerulus;
- renal blood flow;
- the extent of drug protein binding.

The glomerular filtration rate increases with renal blood flow and decreases with increased protein binding of a drug. At birth there is significant anatomical and functional immaturity of the renal tubules.

- Renal blood flow reaches adult levels by the age of 3–5 months.
- The glomerular filtration rate increases considerably from birth, reaching adult levels at 3–5 months.
- Renal function is mature by about 1–3 years of age.

Tubular secretory function does not mature at the same rate as the glomerular filtration rate, as the proximal convoluted tubules are small at birth in relation to the corresponding glomerulus. Adult values of tubular secretion are not reached until about 1 year of age, which affects the elimination of drugs that rely on tubular secretion. The neonate's renal tubules have a smaller surface area and a reduced ability to concentrate urine, with a lower pH compared to infants and older children. The renal function of premature babies and neonates is very poor, which means they excrete drugs very inefficiently. For this reason medicine doses are given much less frequently.

In some clinical conditions, renal clearance can be increased. For example, in cystic fibrosis renal clearance of the antibiotics gentamicin, amikacin, netilimicin and tobramycin is increased and higher doses are often required.

The following activity is to enable you to reflect on and be aware of the extended interval dosing of drugs in premature infants.

Activity 4.7   *Critical thinking*

- Abigail is 5 days old, was born at 28 weeks gestational age and weighs 1,077 grams. She has been prescribed gentamicin for neonatal sepsis.
- Archie is 5 days old, was born at 32 weeks gestational age, weighs 1,644 grams and has also been prescribed gentamicin for a serious infection.

By referring to the *BNF for Children*, calculate the correct prescribed dose for both Abigail and Archie and the dosage interval.

Can you explain the reason for the interval between doses? How does the dose per kilogram compare between a preterm infant and a 1-month-old full-term baby?

Outline answers are provided at the end of the chapter.

Drug dosage and blood levels

Effective drug therapy will only be achieved if the dose of the drug produces the most advantageous concentrations of the drug in the blood plasma and target tissue. The faster the metabolism and excretion of a drug, the less time the drug will remain in the circulation to be available to the tissues. Drugs that are rapidly metabolised and excreted will therefore need to be administered more frequently. A drug's half-life is the time it takes for the plasma concentration of the drug to reach half of its original concentration. The half-life of a drug is therefore how long it takes for half of it to be eliminated from the bloodstream. In order to establish the half-life of a drug, a single dose is given, usually intravenously, and the concentration in the plasma measured at regular intervals. The concentration of the drug will reach a peak level, and then fall as it is cleared from the blood. The time taken for the plasma concentration to halve is the half-life.

For example, if the blood concentration of a drug is 10mg/l at a certain time and this drops to 5mg/l after four hours, then the drug's half-life is four hours. The blood levels would continue to halve every four hours, so would be 2.5 mg/l after two half-lives, 1.25mg/l after three half-lives, 0.625mg/l after four half-lives and 0.3125 mg/l after five half-lives. Therefore, most of a drug is eliminated in five half-lives, regardless of the dose or the route of administration. This rule is used to calculate how long is required from discontinuing one drug and starting another to avoid them interacting with each other.

Some medicines, such as ibuprofen and paracetamol, have very short half-lives (about two hours) and therefore need to be given at regular doses to build up and maintain a high enough concentration in the blood to be effective. Other drugs such as phenobarbital have a much longer half-life (about five days) and take much longer to be eliminated from the plasma, resulting in less frequent dosing. Plasma concentration of a drug will build up with repeated doses until what is known as a steady state is reached (see Figure 4.3).

The steady state is when the amount of drug in the plasma has built up to a concentration level that is therapeutically effective. As long as the drug continues to be administered in regular doses to balance the amount being cleared, the drug will continue to have a therapeutic effect. The time taken to reach the steady state is about five times the half-life of a drug. The intention is to reach a steady-state concentration of a drug during therapy. Drugs that have long half-lives, for example 48 hours, would take ten days to achieve steady state, and drugs with short half-lives of two hours would take less than a day. Long half-lives can be problematic, and sometimes a **loading dose** is administered so that a steady state is reached more quickly, and then smaller **maintenance doses** are given to ensure that the drug levels stay within the steady state. Remember that half-lives will vary from individual to individual and will be affected by the age and weight of the child.

Effective dose/toxic dose

The aim of drug therapy is to ensure that the concentration of drug in the blood is high enough to have a therapeutic effect, but not too high as to have a toxic effect. For all drugs there is a minimum effective concentration below which there will be no therapeutic effect. There is also a concentration of drug in the plasma that, if exceeded, will result in toxicity. This is called the maximum safe concentration. It is important for most drugs that the concentration of the drug in the blood does not fall below the minimum effective concentration. This is the reason why

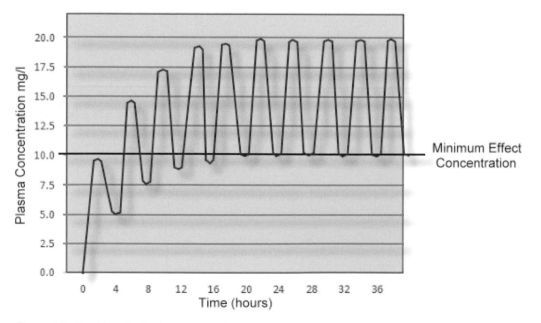

Figure 4.3: Reaching steady-state concentration

drugs should be administered at regular intervals once the steady state has been achieved. Drugs that have a wide gap between maximum and minimum therapeutic concentration are generally safer. This is referred to as the **therapeutic index** (see Figure 4.4). Penicillin is a drug that has such a high therapeutic index that the normal doses given are probably much higher than is actually needed to achieve a therapeutic effect. Some drugs have a low therapeutic index and need to have their plasma levels monitored to ensure that toxic levels are not reached. Examples of drugs with a narrow therapeutic index are gentamicin, warfarin, phenytoin, phenobarbital and digoxin.

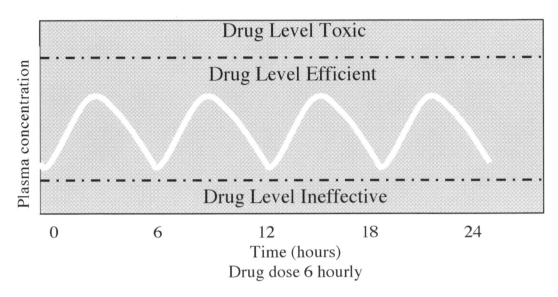

Figure 4.4: The therapeutic index of a drug that is administered every 6 hours

The following activity is to enable you to reflect on and be aware of the need for careful monitoring of plasma concentrations when drugs have a narrow therapeutic index.

Activity 4.8 — *Communication*

Jacey is 13 years old and has been taking 150mg of phenytoin twice daily for the control of tonic-clonic seizures. Her symptoms have recently worsened and she is having more frequent seizures, despite adherence to her medication. The doctor has requested a blood test to measure her plasma–phenytoin concentration. Jacey's father has asked you, as her nurse, why you don't just increase Jacey's phenytoin.

- What is the reason for the blood test before doing this?
- What will you tell the father?

Outline answers are provided at the end of the chapter.

Pharmacodynamics

Pharmacodynamics is the mechanism whereby drugs exert their effects on the body, that is, what the drug does to the body which has a therapeutic effect. Drugs exert their effects in a number of different ways. Those drugs that are a replacement for a deficiency, such as iron, insulin, thyroxine and electrolytes, will act by bringing about a normal physiological response. Other medicines work by having a direct chemical action on the body, such as antacids, which have a chemical reaction with the acid in the stomach and neutralise it. A few drugs, such as simethicone (used for infantile colic), have a physical action. Simethicone is thought to provide a protective coating to the gut wall. Anaesthetic inhalants act by altering the lipid part of cell membranes, resulting in a change in the movement of ions. This causes a change in nerve cell responsiveness, leading to a loss of consciousness.

Other drugs act on specific receptor sites on the cell membrane or in the cell's cytoplasm or nucleus (see Figure 4.5). This is very similar to putting a key in a lock. When a drug binds to a specific receptor it can have an effect on the cell in one of two ways. It can direct an activity within the cell (this type of drug is a receptor agonist). An example of this is salbutamol, which binds with the Beta 2-adrenoreceptor of the smooth muscle in the lungs causing bronchodilation. The second type of effect is when a drug binds with a receptor and thus prevents a naturally occurring substance within the body from binding with it. In this way the normal physiological response is blocked (this type of drug is a receptor antagonist). An example of this is an antihistamine such as cetirizine, which binds to the histamine receptors in the cells to block the action of histamine.

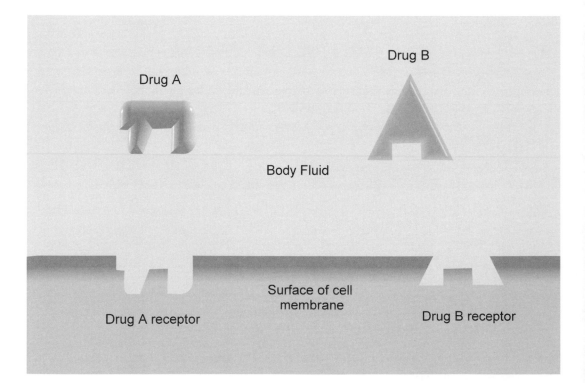

Figure 4.5: Drugs and drug receptors on the cell wall

Drug interactions

Drugs are chemicals and, as such, will interact with each other. When drugs interact with each other, their effects may be rendered inactive or may become suppressed or enhanced. Interactions can occur between drugs at any stage, even before administration, if mixed together in an infusion. It is recommended that drugs are not mixed together before administration in case there is a reaction between them. If many medicines are administered at the same time, the potential for interactions is much higher. It is therefore important that you consult the *BNF for Children* (BMA et al., 2010) for known drug interactions before administration. However, it is impossible to be aware of all the possible interactions, so the children's nurse must be attentive for any possible symptoms of medicine side effects and stop drug therapies immediately and report them. Pharmacokinetic interactions occur when one drug alters the absorption, distribution, protein binding, metabolism or excretion of another. The interaction will reduce or increase the amount of drug available to produce a pharmacological effect.

Absorption

The absorption of drugs may be impaired when other drugs alter the pH of the stomach (antacids) or alter gastrointestinal transit times. Delayed absorption is not usually of clinical importance unless you require quick absorption, for example when giving analgesia (BMA et al., 2010).

Protein binding

Many drugs bind to plasma proteins, in particular albumin. Protein displacement interactions occur when two drugs compete for the same plasma protein, causing one or both drugs to be displaced. This increases the plasma concentration of the free drug. The effect of the increase is often short-lived and compensated for as the increased plasma concentration will result in increased excretion. Exceptions to this are when drugs have a narrow therapeutic margin, or where excretion is delayed due to renal or hepatic impairment.

Metabolism

Some drugs will increase the level of particular enzymes involved in metabolism. Drugs metabolised by this particular enzyme will therefore be broken down more quickly. An example of this is rifampicin, which induces an increase in the enzyme that metabolises oestrogens and progestogens (in the contraceptive pill), resulting in an increased risk of pregnancy. This is the reason women are advised to use an additional form of contraception (such as a condom) when they are prescribed certain antibiotics.

Renal excretion

Competition can occur between drugs for tubular excretion. Some drugs can delay the excretion of others, leading to increased plasma levels and risk of toxicity.

Food

Some foods will react with drugs; one of the most common previously mentioned is the interaction between calcium in food and tetracycline. To avoid this interaction, tetracycline should be taken an hour before, or two hours after, food. Some drugs will prevent the absorption of fat-soluble vitamins in the gastrointestinal tract, and for this reason some children will require vitamin supplementation. One of the most common problems with drug treatment is the effect of the broad spectrum antibiotics on the normal gut flora of the small intestine.

You will find a list of drug interactions in the Appendix of the *BNF for Children* (BMA et al., 2010).

Chapter summary

This chapter has highlighted how children absorb, distribute, metabolise and excrete drugs differently from adults due to their developmental and physiological differences. Absorption of drugs orally will be affected by gastric pH and gastric emptying times. Drugs are metabolised in the body by various organs, but principally the liver. In children, liver enzyme activity may differ compared to adults. Drugs are excreted from the body by numerous routes, but principally by the kidneys, and in premature babies and neonates renal excretion of drugs is inefficient. Body composition in relation to water, extracellular fluid and body fat differs greatly in children and will affect the distribution of drugs in the body. Drug interactions include drug with drug, drug with food and drug with disease. The children's nurse must be knowledgeable and aware of the needs of different age groups of children in relation to medicines management.

Activities: brief outline answers

Activity 4.1 Topical anaesthetics (page 92)

It is easy to forget that a topical cream such as EMLA is a potentially harmful drug. Rapid and extensive absorption can result in systemic side effects so it should be used with caution. EMLA cream is not licensed for use in children less than 1 year old. The dosage instructions for a child aged 1–3 months is to apply a maximum of 1g (tubes generally contain 5g) under occlusive dressing for a maximum of 1 hour before the procedure, maximum one dose in 24 hours. For the child of 1–18 years, apply a thick layer under an occlusive dressing 1–5 hours before the procedure, maximum two doses in 24 hours for child of 1–12 years. The reason for this smaller dose, and shorter application time, is that the cream is being applied to a relatively much larger surface area in the 1–3 month old than the older child. We know that more drug is absorbed systemically the larger the surface area it is applied to and the longer the duration for which it is applied. Also, the drug will be absorbed more easily in the 1–3 month infant, as the stratum corneum of the skin is much thinner.

Activity 4.2 Rectal dose of paracetamol (page 93)

Lydia has been prescribed the correct dose of 500mg for her age and weight orally. As she is vomiting, the preferred route for safety would be rectally and the rectal dose is exactly the same as the oral dose, which is 500mg every 4–6 hours (maximum four doses in 24 hours). However, it is not surprising that, at 12 years of age, Lydia finds the rectal route unacceptable and refuses to give consent. It is fortunate in this situation that intravenous access is available, and although not the safest route it is possible to administer the paracetamol intravenously if the prescriber is willing to prescribe it intravenously. The correct dose for intravenous paracetamol for a child of 10–50kg is 15mg/kg every 4–6 hours (maximum 60mg/kg daily). As Lydia weighs 39kg, the dose would be calculated as $39 \times 15 = 585$mg. The dose must be administered via an intravenous infusion over 15 minutes. Another consideration for the nurse in the management of medicines is drug costs. The cost of the intravenous paracetamol would be approximately £1.50 (plus the cost of any dilutant and the syringe). A 500mg paracetamol tablet would cost less than 5p, and a 500mg suppository would cost about £1.

Activity 4.3 Morphine dosages (page 93)

The correct oral and rectal dose for Michael would be 5–20mg every 4 hours, adjusted according to response. The intravenous dose is 2.5mg–10mg initially over at least five minutes (half the oral dose), and then 2–30 micrograms/kg/hour adjusted according to response. This would be calculated as $50 \times 20 = 100$ micrograms per hour for Michael, much less than the oral dose of more than 5mg every 4 hours. As previously stated, morphine undergoes extensive first pass metabolism by the liver if given orally or rectally, so the bioavailability is greatly reduced. Therefore, the oral and rectal doses need to be much higher than the intravenous dose, which has 100 per cent bioavailability, to compensate for this. Again, the intramuscular dose is 2.5–10mg for Michael, less than for the oral route due to bioavailability being higher.

Activity 4.4 Breastfeeding (page 98)

It is important to encourage Joel's mum to continue breastfeeding as it is much more beneficial nutritionally and immunologically than formula milk. Most medicines taken by breastfeeding mothers cause no harm to breastfed infants and there are few indications to advise a mother to stop breastfeeding because she is taking medication. If you refer to the BNFC and look up 'warfarin', you will notice under the heading 'Cautions' that it states that warfarin is not excreted in breast milk and there is no evidence of harm. You will therefore have the necessary information to reassure Joel's mum that she is safe to continue breastfeeding.

The BNFC identifies those drugs that are contraindicated or should be used with caution when breast-feeding. If a drug is contraindicated, the prescriber will usually try to find a safe alternative. If no safe alternative is available, you could encourage the mother to keep expressing her milk while taking the medication to maintain lactation. She should dispose of the unsafe milk, while temporarily substituting with formula until the medication is completed.

Activity 4.5 Safety of tetracycline (page 99)

Tetracycline is a broad-spectrum antibiotic that can be used in respiratory mycoplasma infection, but it is not licensed for children under 12 years because it can cause discolouration of the teeth. The drug can interact with milk, and Tamara would probably have difficulty swallowing the large tablets (as it is not generally used in children there is no liquid formulation). There are many suitable alternatives for Tamara, such as erythromycin or clarithromycin, so the drug and dosage form should be changed.

Activity 4.6 Drug dosages for an obese child (page 100)

Unfortunately, limited research has been conducted in obese children, so prescribing information is limited. If Bertie was to be prescribed drugs according to his weight, it may result in him receiving much higher doses than necessary, which could be potentially toxic. As a general rule it is advised that the dose should be calculated according to Bertie's ideal weight according to his age and height. (There is a weight/height chart available in the back of the BNFC.) The calculated dose should never be more than an adult dose. Bertie's ideal weight for his height would be 23kg, and the dose should be calculated accordingly.

If in doubt, and where optimal therapeutic doses are essential, it is advised to consult a paediatric pharmacist. Obesity alters the distribution of drugs in the body and this should be taken into consideration. Failure to adjust the dose may result in suboptimal therapy or drug toxicity. Lipophilic drugs may have increased distribution to fatty tissue, thereby decreasing plasma volume and leading to subtherapeutic plasma levels. Also, plasma proteins are altered in obesity, leading to increased binding with some drugs and complicating therapy further.

Activity 4.7 Excretion (page 103)

- The dose for Abigail as a neonate of less than 32 weeks gestational age is 4–5mg/kg every 36 hours (1077 × 4 = 4.308mg every 36 hours).
- The dose for Archie as a neonate over 32 weeks gestational age is the same, 4–5mg/kg; however, the dosage interval is every 24 hours (1644 × 4 = 6.576mg every 24 hours).

Gentamicin is cleared from the body by excretion from the kidneys. The younger the infant, the less developed the kidneys are to excrete the drug. The levels of gentamicin would therefore stay higher in the blood for longer. You will notice in the BNFC also, that the dose for a 1-month-old infant is 2.5mg/kg every 8 hours. The reason for the higher dose per kg in the preterm infant is that gentamicin is a drug that is distributed in water. The preterm infant has a higher percentage of water to body weight, so the drug is more dispersed throughout the body and requires a higher dose per kg weight.

Activity 4.8 Plasma–phenytoin concentration (page 105)

The blood test has been ordered to measure and monitor the amount of phenytoin in the blood and to determine if the drug concentration is within a therapeutic range. If the levels are low, this might be the reason for the increase in Jacey's seizures. A few missed doses or a small change in the drug absorption may have resulted in a marked change in the plasma concentration. Jacey is growing, so the doctor may need to increase the dose. Also, a variety of other drugs, OTC medications and alcohol can interfere with concentrations of phenytoin in the blood. Phenytoin has a very narrow therapeutic index, and a small dose increase in some children can cause a disproportional rise in plasma concentration leading to toxic effects. The doctor must closely monitor the plasma concentration, sometimes daily, to adjust the dose safely.

Further reading

Galbraith, A, Bullock, S, Manias, E, Hunt, B and Richards, A (2007) *Fundamentals of Pharmacology: An applied approach for nursing and health*, 2nd edition. Harlow: Pearson Education.

This text contains numerous learning tools to help you to increase your understanding of pharmacology and apply your knowledge to nursing practice.

Another area for further reading is in the development of pharmacogenetics. Pharmacogenetics examines the role of heredity and response to medicines. It is possible that, in the future, drug therapy may be customised to match a child's genetic make-up.

Useful websites

http://nursingpharmacology.info

This is a nursing pharmacology website with disease-based integrated teaching resources.

Chapter 5
Storing, ordering and receiving medicines in children's nursing

NMC Standards for Pre-registration Nursing Education

This chapter will address the following competencies:

Domain 1: Professional values

1. All nurses must practise with confidence according to *The Code: Standards of conduct, performance and ethics for nurses and midwives* (NMC, 2008), and within other recognised ethical and legal frameworks. They must be able to recognise and address ethical challenges relating to people's choices and decision-making about their care, and act within the law to help them and their families and carers find acceptable solutions.

NMC Essential Skills Clusters

This chapter will address the following ESCs:

Cluster: Medicines management

37. People can trust the newly registered graduate nurse to safely order, receive, store and dispose of medicines (including controlled drugs) in any setting.

By the second progression point:

1. Demonstrates ability to safely store medicines under supervision.

By entry to the register:

2. Orders, receives, stores and disposes of medicines safely (including controlled drugs).

Chapter aims

By the end of this chapter, you should be able to:

* understand the legislation that underpins practice in relation to the ordering and storing of medicines, such as controlled drugs, infusions and oxygen;
* describe how to manage medicines, both in hospital and in primary care settings such as schools and patients' homes;
* identify suitable conditions for storage and management of out-of-date stock, manage discrepancies and omissions in stock and safely handle medicines.

Case study

It was widely reported in 1997 that an 11-year-old boy had died, two hours after being taken to hospital after suffering a severe asthma attack at school. The boy became breathless at lunchtime but then improved to return to lessons. After experiencing a severe asthmatic attack in his next lesson, he was told to wait in a corridor by a teacher. He was not directed to staff trained in first aid or taken to hospital until his mother arrived at the end of the day. The doctor at the hospital who treated him said that he could have been saved if he had been taken to hospital earlier. There had been a number of failings in the school's medical procedures. The medical records from his primary school and a letter from his doctor had not been added to his school journal, or the school's online information system.

This case highlights the need for children to have immediate access to their medicines in schools and other settings. The boy had suffered from asthma all his life, and would have undoubtedly needed access to his asthma medication during his school day. The severity of his asthma should have prompted a care planning meeting in the school between parents, teachers and the school nurse for a written care plan to be agreed. The school staff did not appear to know what to do in the event of an asthma attack. It also shows the need for good record keeping, communication and staff training in the management of children with complex health needs in schools, in order to prevent such tragedies. School and community nurses have a role to play in liaison with schools on pupils' needs. There are large numbers of children in the UK today attending school with chronic conditions such as asthma, epilepsy, diabetes, cystic fibrosis and severe allergies who require access to medicines and school staff trained in emergencies.

Introduction

All children's nurses at some point in their career will be required to handle medicines. The term 'medicines' includes all products administered orally, topically or internally (including all injections and infusions) for the purpose of treating, diagnosing or preventing disease. This chapter will outline the procedures for the safe handling and storage of medicines in line with national guidance and legislation.

First, we will look at the responsibilities of registered nurses and nurse managers for the safe storage of medicines, and will go on to review good practice for the supply and ordering of medicines, including controlled drugs, both in the community and in hospital settings. Next, we will discuss the safe storage of vaccines, including transportation and the disposal and return of medicines. In the next section, we review the management of cytotoxic drugs, including spillage and waste disposal, and finally we will examine the storage and administration of medicines in schools and other settings.

Your employer must ensure that all medicines are handled and stored in a safe and secure manner.

Security of medicines in storage

The nurse manager or senior nurse is generally responsible for the safekeeping of medicines in their clinical area. From the time a medicine is received until its removal or disposal, it should be kept securely and only authorised personnel should have access to that medicine. All medicine cupboards and refrigerators should be kept locked at all times and the keys kept in a secure place or by an authorised person.

Responsibilities of the registered nurse

As a registered nurse you are responsible for ensuring that you are appropriately trained and aware of current policies and procedures with regard to the safety and security of medicines. You must understand your scope of practice and work within it. You must identify and adhere to the policy of your employer and have an understanding of what documentation you need to complete (NMC, 2010b). As a registered nurse, you are also responsible for safeguarding yourself and those under your care and supervision from any risk posed by medicinal products.

Responsibilities of line managers

It is the responsibility of the department manager to ensure that all employees are trained with regard to the safety and security of medicines, and understand the need for risk management in relation to drug products and procedures. The senior manager may delegate to a health professional the responsibility of ensuring the safe handling and storage of medicines for a specific area.

Classification of medicines and related preparations

As described in Chapter 2, medicines are classified under the Medicines Act 1968 into three main categories, shown in Table 5.1.

Category	Description
Prescription-only medicines (POMs)	These are medicines that may only be supplied or administered to a patient on the instruction of an appropriate practitioner, such as a doctor, dentist or non-medical prescriber.
Pharmacy-only (P) medicines	These can be purchased from a registered primary care pharmacy, provided the pharmacist supervises the sale.
General sales list (GSL) medicines	These need neither a prescription nor the supervision of a pharmacist and can be obtained from retail outlets.

Table 5.1: Classification of medicines

The Misuse of Drugs Act 1971 controls the export, import, production, supply and possession of drugs that are dangerous or otherwise harmful. The use of controlled drugs (CDs) in medicine is permitted under the Misuse of Drugs Regulations 2001(see Chapter 2). Table 5.2 shows the controlled drugs, which are classified under five schedules.

Schedule	Description
Schedule 1 (cannabis, cannabis resin, coca leaf, lysergide)	Schedule 1 drugs have no recognised medicinal use; practitioners may not lawfully possess Schedule 1 drugs unless they have a special licence to do so from the Home Office, for specific purposes such as research.
Schedule 2 (CD POMs) (methadone, morphine, cocaine, diamorphine)	Schedule 2 CDs may be administered to a patient by any person authorised to prescribe them, or by any person acting in accordance with the directions of an appropriate person authorised to prescribe CDs. This includes nurse independent prescribers, who are currently permitted to prescribe, administer and direct others to administer certain CDs for specific conditions and routes of administration.
Schedule 3 (temazepam, buprenorphine, phentermine) (CD No Register)	Schedule 3 includes drugs such as minor stimulants that are thought to be less likely to be misused, or less harmful when misused than drugs in Schedule 2. Schedule 3 drugs are exempt from safe custody requirements; however, temazepam, flunitrazepam, buprenorphine and diethylpropion are exceptions that must be stored in a CD cupboard in a secure environment.
Schedule 4 (CD benzodiazepines and anabolic steroids) Examples of Schedule 4 drugs, part I: • clonazepam • tetrazepam • nitrazepam Examples of Schedule 4 drugs, part II: • mesterolone • testosterone • nandrolone	Schedule 4 has two parts. In part I are benzodiazepines and other substances, while part II contains anabolic steroids and androgenic steroids, as well as other substances. It is an offence to possess a drug from Schedule 4, part I, without an appropriate prescription. There is no restriction on the possession of a part II CD anabolic steroid drug when it is part of a medicinal product.

Table 5.2: Controlled drugs

Schedule	Description
Schedule 5 (CD Invoice) Examples of Schedule 5 drugs: • preparations containing not more than 0.1% cocaine • preparations containing not more than 0.2% morphine	These are preparations that contain low strengths of certain CDs such as codeine and morphine, but are exempt from full control as the risk of misuse is reduced. There are no restrictions on their possession, import, export or administration or destruction, and safe custody regulations do not apply. However, invoices for these preparations must be kept for at least two years.

Table 5.2: Continued

The medicine trail

To ensure safe and secure handling of medicines within organisations there must be systems in place to facilitate auditing of transactions from purchase and supply to the disposal of any waste product. This system is often referred to as the **medicine trail**.

The procurement of medicines

Procurement is the term applied to the acquisition of medicines for the purpose of treating a patient, and must comply with current legislation and any financial restrictions. The procurement of medicines can take place by various routes, but the principles of procurement remain the same throughout individual settings.

Medicines dispensing and supply arrangements

Dispensing medicines to patients from pharmacies is the preferred model of practice for patient safety and effectiveness. Dispensing and other supply arrangements outside pharmacies, such as clinics and walk-in centres, must be developed in conjunction with the local pharmacies and authorised by the **Chief Pharmacist** and endorsed by the local **Medicines Management Committee**.

The supply and ordering of medicines

The senior nurse has overall responsibility for the nursing supplies cupboard's contents. A list of all medicines and their stock list for the specific area is held and decided following consultation with the local Medicines Management Committee and is usually subject to annual review.

The medicines and other preparations are usually supplied through a regular top-up service by the local pharmacy supplier. When stocks are running low between the top-up service, the ordering of medicines can be delegated to another member of staff, such as clerical staff, but it usually remains the responsibility of the senior nurse to assess what needs to be ordered.

Stock checking and ordering should take place at regular intervals, appropriate to the needs of the service, which would probably be on a weekly basis or at least two-weekly. Official order forms should be stored safely in a locked cupboard and medicines should only be supplied on the instruction of an authorised signatory. The order form should include the date and name of the person placing the order, and a copy is kept to check against the delivery note. Telephone orders are not normally acceptable. Delivery records should normally be kept for a period of two years as a record that the medicines were supplied. Practitioners carrying out regular stock checks are responsible for reporting any discrepancies to the nurse manager. Nurses are responsible for ensuring that the medicines cupboard is kept clean and tidy to allow for easy stock checking and top-up.

Scenario

Mark is a registered children's nurse in a busy children's walk-in centre. It is Friday morning and Mark is dispensing a 100mL bottle of paracetamol oral suspension under a PGD. When Mark looks in the medicine cupboard, he notices that there are only two more bottles of paracetamol oral suspension there. This concerns Mark as he is aware that the walk-in centre will require more than two bottles to last over the weekend. Mark informs his nursing manager, Alison, who telephones the pharmacy to ask why they have not been stocked up. The pharmacy confirms that there was a delay in restocking this week due to staff sickness, but they will deliver some stock today to ensure that enough is available for the weekend.

It is the responsibility of all practitioners to ensure that stock levels are appropriately managed.

The emergency supply of medicines

The emergency supply of medicines (such as a telephone consultation on a Friday evening with a patient who has run out of their regular medication) should only take place if it would be harmful to the patient to delay administration of the medicine until a signed prescription is made available. The doctor should contact the pharmacy and ask them to supply the medicine; the doctor requesting the emergency supply must attend and sign a relevant prescription as soon as is reasonably practicable, or within 24 hours. It is considered acceptable for a facsimile of the prescription to be sent to the pharmacy to avoid delay. The emergency supply of controlled drugs is not acceptable.

Scenario

Sarah is a registered nurse providing telephone triage for a GP out-of-hours service. She receives a telephone call on Friday evening at seven o'clock from Mick, the father of 6-year-old James. Mick explains that he is very

continued opposite . . .

continued . . .

worried as he has no asthma medication for the weekend for James. Mick is separated from James's mother and it is his turn to have James with him over the weekend. He has just checked James's bag and noticed that his asthma reliever medication has run out. Mick telephoned James's mother, who informed him she had forgotten to order a repeat prescription. Mick knows that he will definitely need to give James his reliever over the weekend as he often gets wheezy when he is staying with him.

Sarah is very understanding and feels that a delay in receiving the asthma reliever could be harmful to James. Sarah contacts the doctor covering the service, who telephones Mick's local pharmacy to request an emergency supply of the medication. The doctor then sends a facsimile of the prescription to ensure that the correct dose and formula are dispensed. The pharmacist agrees to the prescription being delivered by the doctor at a convenient time on Saturday.

The emergency supply of the asthma reliever possibly avoided James experiencing an exacerbation of his asthma and an attendance at the accident and emergency department.

Ordering controlled drugs

Following a 2007 Home Office-led review and public consultation, changes were made to the Misuse of Drugs Regulations 2001 and the Misuse of Drugs Regulations (Northern Ireland) 2002. These changes affect the requirements for requisitions for CDs in the community in order to safeguard against the risk of diversion and abuse of the supply of CDs. The changes do not apply to supplies from NHS hospital trusts, care homes and pharmaceutical wholesalers, as present procedures are considered adequate for the care and safe handling in these organisations. From January 2008 it is a legal requirement that all CD requisition forms completed by practitioners are stored for a period of two years to allow for their retrieval. Dedicated requisition forms were introduced for the supply of controlled drugs in the community, which are readily distinguishable and include a unique serial number to identify the profession of the practitioner ordering the CD.

The senior nurse is usually responsible for the order, receipt and storage of CDs, which can only be ordered from a pharmacy by submitting a requisition from the CD requisition book in line with legislation. All CDs must be delivered to the premises and received by a registered practitioner who must sign for the secure package on the drugs delivery record sheet. The registered practitioner must check the amount delivered against the requisition and, if correct, sign the requisition. If there are any discrepancies, they should be reported to the pharmacy and manager immediately. The registered practitioner must enter the new stock in the CD record book on the appropriate page, witnessed by another registered practitioner, who must also verify the stock levels and sign the record book. If sealed tamper-proof packs of drugs are supplied, it is not necessary to open these packs for stock checking purposes. The CDs must be immediately locked away in a controlled medicines cupboard, access to which is restricted to registered practitioners. All CD record and requisition books are controlled stationery, only available from a medicines management team, and should always be locked away to prevent tampering. All orders and records must be completed in permanent ink and must be retained for two years from the last entry in the book. If a discrepancy occurs between the stock balance and the CD record book, the nurse in charge must inform the senior manager immediately.

> ### Scenario
>
> *Gayle is a registered children's nurse working in a community hospice. She is completing the daily check of CDs with another registered nurse and recording the findings in the CD record book. Gayle and her colleague notice that there is a discrepancy between the stock balance of Oramorph oral solution and the record book. They are unable to account for 200mL of the oral solution. They check the ward stock and the prescriptions of all the patients prescribed Oramorph, but it is still unaccounted for. Gayle immediately informs the hospice manager who is the accountable officer (AO) for the hospice. The AO for the hospice is responsible for contacting the AO in the PCT to organise an incident panel to investigate the discrepancy and then, if necessary, contact the police.*
>
> *Simon, the hospice nurse manager and AO, arrives. Gayle and Simon search the other medicine cupboards and discover that the 200mL of Oramorph had been placed in another medicines cupboard. An incident form is completed with all the information and Simon establishes which nurses were on duty when this occurred. It is possible that this was an innocent error; however, it could have been an attempt to acquire a CD for personal use by a member of staff. An audit of CD use, order, delivery, receipt and stock is undertaken to try to identify any errors. Gayle and her colleague were reassured by the manager that they acted appropriately and were thanked.*

Receipt of medicines

All medicines received by wards or community premises should be delivered by the relevant pharmacy supplier in a securely locked and sealed box. If they are not, this should be reported to the supplier for investigation. Medicines received should be checked for quantity and quality, and signed for by the senior nurse or nurse in charge. If a registered nurse is not available, a responsible member of staff can sign for the delivery (with the exception of CDs). The sealed box must then be stored in a locked cupboard until the registered nurse or practitioner is available to receive the supply. Medicines should be removed from the sealed delivery receptacle and stored in the appropriate medicines cupboard as soon as possible within the working day. Items for refrigeration are transported in cool boxes and are identified to be placed in the refrigerator immediately on receipt. A responsible member of staff may do this on behalf of the senior nurse or nurse in charge. Again, the order must be checked against the delivery note and signed for, noting any discrepancies and reporting any to the pharmacy supplier.

Stock rotation

Stock rotation is an important aspect of medicines management, and expiry dates of existing stock must be checked and stock with the shortest expiry date used first. Expired stock must be removed from the cupboard and returned to the supplier after completion of a 'returned medicines' form.

Storage of medicines

The stock level of medicines stored in any clinical area will generally be subject to continuous audit and changes made accordingly by medicines management leads. All medicines stored should always remain in the manufacturers' original packaging and must be stored in locked cupboards, which should be reserved solely for the storage of medicinal products, in order to ensure the safety of patients and staff. The nurse in charge is responsible for holding and storing the keys, which should be clearly identified and kept on a separate key ring. A secure system for access to the keys should be established between those practitioners authorised to use them. The area designated for medicines storage should not be accessible to the public, and any breach in this security should be reported immediately to the lead nurse. Cupboards designated for medicines storage should comply with British Standards. It is also recommended for the purpose of safety that medicines are separated into different locked cupboards for storage according to whether they are:

- medicines for internal use – tablets, elixirs, injections;
- medicines for external use – ointments, creams, dressings;
- refrigerated items;
- controlled drugs;
- disinfectants and antiseptics;
- clinical reagents;
- baby milks.

Separate sections are required within the cupboards and refrigerators to segregate the different categories of drugs, such as oral preparations from injections. Stocks should be checked regularly to ensure all products are still within their expiry date and are free from damage. Medicines must be protected from contamination and damage from exposure to sunlight, moisture and adverse temperatures. Any damaged or expired stock must be returned to the pharmacy supplier and recorded on a returned medicines form. Samples of medicines or dressings should not be accepted from pharmaceutical representatives for storage in clinics or use on patients.

Scenario

Debbie is a community children's nurse who has been asked to run a new vaccination clinic in a remote GP surgery. On arrival, the receptionist directs Debbie to the drug fridge where the vaccines are stored. Debbie notices that the fridge in the clinic room is not locked, and that there are stool and urine specimens being stored alongside the vaccines. Debbie asks the receptionist if this usually happens, and is told that they have always kept patient specimens in the same fridge and often keep their sandwiches in there also. Debbie immediately informs the practice manager that this practice is not acceptable under the law and the specimens need to be removed. The fridge must be locked and kept in a lockable room. If the fridge is constantly being opened, the drop in temperature could degrade the vaccines. It is also not good infection control practice to keep potentially contaminated specimens and food next to vaccines.

Emergency drugs

Medicines for clinical emergencies should be marked clearly 'for emergency use' and stored so that practitioners can access them easily during clinic sessions. They must remain in their sealed containers so that they have clearly not been tampered with, and once seals are broken they must be replaced. They should be secured in the same way as other drugs when clinics are not in use.

Controlled drugs

Controlled drugs must always be stored in accordance with the Misuse of Drugs (Safe Custody) Regulations 1973. They must be stored in a locked cabinet in a lockable room that is not accessible to patients. The keys to the lockable cabinet are the responsibility of the registered nurse in charge and must be kept separate from the cabinet. It is usual for there to be one set of keys only; the number of sets of keys and who holds them must be known at all times.

Only the registered nurse in charge or a person authorised by them should open the cabinet, the nurse in charge remaining ultimately responsible. The CD record book, listing the stock levels of the cabinet, should be kept in an appropriate location outside the cabinet.

Activity 5.1   *Team working*

You are the nurse in charge of an out-of-hours clinic and the doctor on duty asks you for the keys to the CD cupboard so that he can administer pethidine to a patient.

- What action should you take?

An outline answer is provided at the end of the chapter.

Medicines refrigerators

Refrigerators used to store medicines and vaccines should be designed for the purpose, with uniform temperature throughout; domestic models are not suitable. The refrigerator must be lockable in accordance with Control of Substances Hazardous to Health (COSHH) Regulations, and have proper safeguards against power failure if used for storing vaccines. The refrigerator should have a minimum–maximum thermometer and the temperature should be monitored daily. The medicines refrigerator should be used specifically for the storage of medicines or vaccines and not for other items, such as patients' specimens. The fridge should be lockable and should be kept within a lockable room. All medicines received should be checked for storage instructions and medicines requiring storage below room temperature will be clearly marked 'store in a refrigerator between 2 and 8 degrees centigrade'.

There is more information about vaccines and their storage in the following section.

Prescription pads

All prescription pads should be kept in a securely locked cupboard in a locked room and a record of the serial numbers should be kept separately in case of loss or theft. The security of prescription pads in use is the responsibility of the medical or non-medical prescriber. The organisation's prescribing lead is responsible for the ordering, distribution and recording of serial numbers.

Medicines storage in patients' homes

All nurses should advise parents, grandparents, children and young people on the safe storage and handling of medicines in the home. Advice should include storing medicines in a secure place, away from children, and avoiding extremes of temperature, sunlight and humidity. All medicines, tablets, vitamins and herbal remedies should be locked in a medicine cabinet or other cupboard so that children cannot access them.

Children have a natural curiosity and young children are often tempted to try medicines that adults have left in the bedroom, bathroom or kitchen. Medicine poisoning can be very serious and many children are admitted to accident and emergency departments with suspected poisoning by medicines. Many of these accidental poisonings occur when young children are visiting a grandparent or relative who is not used to having to lock medicines away. Always remind adults to keep medicines out of children's reach.

The storage of methadone

Accidental poisoning by methadone can be fatal and can occur as a result of children ingesting a parent's methadone. An audit by Mullin et al. (2008) found serious concerns regarding the storage of methadone in the home and identified this as a risk to families. Of patients who were prescribed methadone and stored it at home, 60 per cent had children either living with them or visiting the home. The patients' recall of being given information about safety was poor. Nurses have a responsibility to ensure that parents using methadone are given verbal and written information and guidance on safe storage in order to protect children from accidental ingestion.

The transportation of medicines

As a registered nurse you have a duty of care to take all reasonable steps to ensure the security at all times of any medicines that you have in your possession. You should not transfer medicines between sites unless in exceptional circumstances and, if you do so, all transfers must be recorded. Medicines transferred between sites should be carried in locked, security-sealed containers. If you receive stock from another site not in a security-sealed container, you must document and report this immediately to your manager for investigation.

Community nurses

As a community children's nurse you should not collect patients' prescriptions from community pharmacies under normal circumstances. Parents and families should collect their own prescriptions, and when this is not possible most pharmacies now operate a home delivery service. Only under exceptional circumstances, such as an emergency, should a community nurse transport controlled or prescription-only drugs in their own car. Where medicines are transported in a car, they should be carried directly to the patient, securely locked in the boot of the car. You should also be aware of extremes of temperatures that may affect the drug, in particular drugs such as vaccines, which should be transported in a cool box.

The use and storage of medical gases

All cylinders containing medical gases (oxygen, Entonox and nitrous oxide) should be stored in a secure area in order to prevent unauthorised access and to protect cylinders from theft. They should be firmly secured with safety chains or a stand to prevent them falling over. The number of cylinders kept as stock in the clinical area should be kept to a minimum.

Cylinders containing different gases should be separated within the store, which should be indoors and not subject to heat or cold. Warning notices should be posted, prohibiting smoking and naked lights, within the vicinity of medical gases, and oil or grease should never be applied to the cylinder or connectors. Cylinders with the oldest filling date should be used first and, when empty, placed separately from full cylinders so that they can be collected and replaced by the supplier.

Excessive force or tools should not be used for opening or closing the cylinder valves, and cylinders with damaged valves or defects should be labelled as damaged and withdrawn from use.

The fire service should be informed of the location and contents of any medical gases stored in the community or in patients' homes.

Oxygen management in the community

Many children are now being discharged home on oxygen therapy and it is essential that they receive all the necessary equipment and supplies they need. The pharmacy supplier of the oxygen has a duty to ensure that parents or others operating the equipment are supported and educated in its safe use. Community children's nurses should be aware of the local policies and procedures for the provision, replacement and repair of equipment. Each child should have a management plan in which the amount of oxygen that can be administered is documented, and the guidelines for the need for admission to hospital. Before discharge, parents should receive training in CPR, which should be documented, and how to recognise a deterioration of symptoms. This is to ensure that parents are able to manage an emergency and can recognise when a child needs medical help. Parents need training in the use of **apnoea monitors** and **oxygen saturation monitors** if they are used, and what to do if they alarm (NMPDU, 2002). There must be access to a telephone in the home for emergency use.

The home storage and transportation of oxygen

Parents need to be aware of the risks posed by oxygen, which is stored in containers under pressure and increases the rate at which things burn once a fire starts. Precautions should be taken to reduce the risks of fire during storage and transport. Oxygen equipment should be stored away from potential sources of combustion. Smoking should not be permitted in any vehicle carrying oxygen or in the home were oxygen is stored.

To prevent damage, cylinders should be strapped or held so that they do not get damaged and should be stored out of direct sunlight (NHS, 2010b). Cylinders should be checked for obvious signs of leaks, such as hissing sounds, before a journey. Vehicle windows should be partially opened when oxygen is being transported and no more than two cylinders should be carried on each journey. A vehicle Transport Emergency (TREM) card should be carried at all times when oxygen is being transported. Parents need to inform their car insurance company that oxygen is being carried in the vehicle. If a child needs to travel with oxygen on public transport, checks need to be made with the transport company for permission to do this. If it is not permitted to travel on local public transport, parents can claim for the costs of taxis or for 'motability' (NMPDU, 2002).

Children using oxygen outside the home will do so through the use of portable cylinders. Parents need to be able to calculate the length of time the cylinder will last, so they need to be provided with oxygen cylinder duration times. A plan of action needs to be devised so that parents know what to do if oxygen runs out and is not available to the child.

The use of oxygen in schools and other settings

It is important that children requiring oxygen therapy are allowed to attend school and other settings to continue their education. The school nurses and paediatrician will need to collaborate with the school or other setting and parents to develop a school healthcare plan to include guidelines for the administration of oxygen. Designated staff need to be instructed on the safe administration of oxygen, such as flow rates, and should be given resuscitation training. The GP would normally supply a prescription for the pharmacy supplier to deliver oxygen cylinders to the school or other setting. Written information regarding safe storage should be provided.

The storage of vaccines

Vaccines are used frequently within children's nursing practice and in the UK include routine childhood vaccines for diphtheria, polio, tetanus, pertussis (whooping cough), Haemophilus influenza type b (Hib), meningitis C (MenC), pneumococcal infections and MMR (measles, mumps and rubella). These vaccines can be administered in community settings, such as Sure Start Children's Centres, and need to be transported and stored. And, at times, vaccines may be administered in the homes of hard-to-reach client groups, such as travellers and poor clinic attendees. Immunisation against human papillomavirus was introduced for girls aged 12–13 years in 2008 and is usually given by school nurses, so has to be transported to school premises.

Vaccines are biological substances and will biodegrade naturally over time and have a predetermined shelf life. The vaccine's expiry date is dependent on correct storage and the vaccine will biodegrade sooner if it is stored outside the recommended temperature range. Incorrect storage of vaccines will lead to a loss of vaccine potency, resulting in a failure of the vaccine to protect the recipient. Allowing vaccines to become too warm or too cold at any time during their storage or transport will also lead to vaccine wastage. Vaccines must be kept at temperatures of between 2 and 8 degrees centigrade and correct temperatures will be indicated on the vaccine packaging.

A log should be kept of all fridge temperature readings on all working days, including time of recording, maximum, minimum and actual temperature. The log should include the name of the person taking the recordings, and any action that resulted from readings outside the safe storage range. The log must be available for inspection by Medicines Management Board staff on request. All clinical areas that order and store vaccines should have a designated person responsible for this, to ensure that stock levels are maintained and stock rotation is practised to avoid wastage. Vaccines required for community settings, such as baby clinics and schools, should be transported in an appropriate cool box to maintain the cold chain and returned to the refrigerator as soon as possible if unused.

Activity 5.2 — *Leadership and management*

You are a school nurse about to carry out a vaccination clinic in one of your schools. You arrive at the community clinic to collect the vaccines and you find the power to the fridge is off as the plug has been pulled out of the socket. You need to start your clinic soon.

*   What will you do?

An outline answer is provided at the end of the chapter.

The disposal and return of medicines

Medicines should never be disposed of in domestic or commercial refuse collection systems and it is illegal to dispose of medicines in the sewerage system, such as flushing them down toilets or sinks. Medicines obtained for a patient on prescription remain the property of the patient and they should not be returned to the ward, clinic or health centre. Parents and patients should be encouraged to return unwanted medicines to their local pharmacy to ensure safe disposal.

Controlled drugs no longer required by patients should also be returned to the local pharmacy to be disposed of in accordance with the local policy for the destruction of CDs.

The return of medicines from community clinics

Medicines received in community clinics that have expired or are unwanted can be returned to the pharmacy supplier as agreed by local policy. This would normally be done as soon as is reasonably practicable. Any out-of-date stock should be removed and stored in a separate locked cupboard for return to avoid erroneous administration. Normally, two copies of a returned medicines form would be completed, one retained by the clinic, the other returned with the medicines in a locked, security-sealed container. The container must be stored in a secure place until collected, and the date of return should be recorded in the appropriate log book. Expired or unwanted CDs must not be returned in this way; the Head of Medicines Management or AO must be contacted so that an authorised person can attend to witness the proper destruction of the stock.

The destruction of expired or unwanted CDs

As mentioned earlier, the Health Act 2006 requires that the designated body (e.g. PCT) appoints an accountable officer (AO) to be responsible for the safe and secure handling of controlled drugs within the organisation. The AO is able to authorise and hold a record of suitable individuals to witness the destruction of controlled drugs. Authorised individuals must not be involved in the daily management of CDs and should be either subject to a professional code of ethics or to Criminal Records Bureau (CRB) checking. The person should be trained to carry out witnessed destructions according to local policy.

The disposal of sharps

The handling of sharps should be kept to a minimum and used sharps disposed of into a designated sharps box. Syringes and needles should not be separated but disposed of as one unit. The sharps box should be labelled with the name of the assembler and the date assembled. Sharps boxes should always be stored in a secure place out of reach of children and should be securely locked once they become three-quarters full.

Cytotoxic medicines

It is essential that precautions are taken when handling cytotoxic medicines, as they have the potential to cause **carcinogenic**, **teratogenic** and **mutagenic** effects. Cytotoxic drugs should never be handled or administered by pregnant women. They may be accidentally absorbed through the skin or by inhalation, and can cause damage to the skin, eyes and mucous membranes. Cytotoxic drugs should not be reconstituted or drawn up in community settings and must be supplied in appropriately labelled ready-to-use pre-filled syringes. Personal protective equipment (PPE) such as gowns, aprons and gloves should be worn according to local risk assessments that should be carried out.

Accidental contact with cytotoxic medicines

Any cytotoxic medicine that accidentally comes into contact with skin should be washed off immediately with soap and water. Any that accidentally comes into contact with the eyes should be immediately rinsed out with water or saline. Occupational Health should be informed of any of the above incidents and the nurse or client should be reviewed by a doctor. An incident form must always be completed and the nurse manager informed.

The management of cytotoxic drug spillage

All sites where cytotoxic drugs are stored or administered must hold a cytotoxic spillage kit in order to deal with any spillage immediately. Plastic aprons and gloves should be worn, along with safety glasses if there is a risk of splashing. Absorbent gauze swabs from the spillage kit should be used to soak up the spilt medicine, and then the area should be cleaned with soap and water, again using the absorbent gauze swabs. All contaminated cleaning materials should then be disposed of in the clinical waste.

Cytotoxic waste

Any sharps, swabs, syringes or other containers that may have come into contact with a cytotoxic drug must be disposed of as cytotoxic waste into a specifically designated cytotoxic waste container.

Activity 5.3   *Team working*

You are the community children's nurse providing palliative care to 3-year-old Amy in her own home. You return after two weeks' leave, during which time a colleague has been visiting the family daily. You notice there is a discrepancy in the amount of morphine that is left when you check the stock before administration.

- What should you do?

An outline answer is provided at the end of the chapter.

The storage and administration of medicines in schools and other settings

Under the Special Educational Needs and Disability Act (SENDA) 2001 and the Disability Discrimination Act (DDA) 1995, children with medical needs who require medication should have the same admission rights to schools and other settings and need to be accommodated. Children with long-term or short-term medical conditions need to be able to continue attending school (including boarding schools) or other settings, and consideration needs to be given as to how their medical needs can be met. These settings could include day-care settings such as nursery schools, childminders' homes, children's centres, breakfast clubs, after-school clubs and holiday clubs. All settings need to comply with health and safety regulations and it is the responsibility of each setting to develop policies and procedures around the management of medicines.

Policy guidelines

Policies should include:

- procedures for managing prescription medicines during the school day;
- procedures for managing medicines on school trips;
- the roles and responsibilities of staff: who will take responsibility for the administration of medicines and its witnessing;
- parents' responsibilities and written agreements;
- staff training;
- procedures for the checking of medication before administration;
- storage;
- record keeping;
- disposal of medicines;
- what to do if a child refuses medication;
- the administration of non-prescription medications;
- information on children carrying their own medicines and self-administration;
- emergency procedures;
- risk assessment.

The administration of medicines

The Medicines Act 1968 places restrictions on the administration of medicinal products within the UK. Where a school or day-care setting agrees to administer any medicines, the employer must ensure that the risks to the health of others are properly controlled. This responsibility is set out in the Control of Substances Hazardous to Health Regulations 2002. Anyone (which can include teachers, teaching assistants etc.) may administer a prescribed medicine to a third party, as long as they have valid consent and the medicine is being administered in accordance with the prescriber's instructions.

Parents should provide schools and other settings with full information about their child's medical needs, including all details of the medicines and their side effects. Written consent should be obtained from parents before administering medicines to children under 16 years. The medicine may only be administered to the person it has been prescribed for and supplied to, and it must be labelled. The member of staff should check the child's name, prescribed dose and the expiry date before administering the dose. No one other than the prescriber is permitted to vary the dose or the directions for administration. This also applies to the injection of prescription-only medicines, as long as the injection is administered in accordance with the directions of the prescriber to a named patient. If staff are in doubt about any procedure, they should not administer the medicine but check with the parents or a health professional.

Controlled drugs

The Misuse of Drugs Regulations 2001 allows 'any person' to administer the drugs listed in the Regulations. This means that it is permissible for someone within a school or day-care setting to administer a CD with consent to a child, as long as it is prescribed and in accordance with the prescriber's directions.

Prescribed medicines

Medicines should only be prescribed for administration during school hours if it would be detrimental to the child's health not to do so. The National Service Framework for Children (Medicines Standard 6) (DH, 2004a) recommends that a range of options are explored by the prescriber to avoid the need for medicines to be taken during school or day-care hours. These options include dose frequencies that need to be administered only once or twice a day, so they can be taken outside school hours. Even medicines that need to be taken three times a day could be taken in the morning, after school and then at bedtime. Parents should be encouraged to discuss this with the prescriber. When necessary, the prescriber may provide two prescriptions for the child's medicine, one for home use and one for school use, avoiding the need to keep transporting the medicine between settings (for example, as-required asthma inhalers).

Non-prescription medicines

In general, non-prescription medicines should not be given to children in schools or other settings unless there is specific prior written consent from the parents to do so. An example of this could be the administration of paracetamol when required for minor ailments, or vitamin supplements in a boarding school setting. The school policy should set out the circumstances under which staff may administer non-prescription medications. Children under 16 years should never be given medicines containing aspirin unless prescribed by a doctor.

Storing medicine in schools and day-care settings

The head or senior staff member is responsible for ensuring that medicines are stored safely.

Only medicines that have been prescribed by a qualified health professional, such as a doctor, dentist, nurse or pharmacist prescriber, should be accepted for storage and administration in schools and day-care settings. The medicine should be properly dispensed by a pharmacist, in the original container, and labelled with the child's name and prescriber's instructions. Medicines should not be accepted if they are not in their original container, and changes cannot be made to the original doses on parental instructions. Schools and day-care settings should not store large volumes of medicines, which should be stored in accordance with the manufacturer's instructions. Medicines that need to be refrigerated can be kept in a refrigerator containing food. However, there should be restricted access to the refrigerator and the medicine should be in a clearly labelled, airtight container. If a child requires more than one prescribed medication, each should be in its original container as dispensed by a pharmacist and never transferred into another container. Children who have Type 1 diabetes should be provided with appropriate fridge space for the storage of insulin and safe storage space for a blood glucose testing kit. They should have access to a clean and private environment and sharps bins for the disposal of needles (RCN, 2009).

Access to medicines

School-age children requiring medication need to have access to their medicines, know where their medicines are and know who holds the key. Medicines that may be required for the management of an emergency situation, such as asthma inhalers and adrenaline pens, should be readily available to children and not locked away. It is policy in many schools to allow children to carry their own asthma inhalers so that they have immediate access to them; however, this policy must be balanced to ensure that only children prescribed the medications have access to them. Non-emergency medicine should in general be kept in a secure place so that it is not accessible to children. Department for Education and Skills standards (DfES, 2003) require that medicines should be stored in their original containers, clearly labelled and inaccessible to children. All schools and day-care settings should make special arrangements for access to medicines during an emergency.

Self-management

The age at which children are ready to be responsible for their own medicines varies with each individual child. It is good practice to support and encourage children to take responsibility for managing their own medicines when they are ready and able to do so. Older children with a long-term medical condition should, in most cases, be able to take complete responsibility for their medicines. Health professionals should assist parents and children to make decisions about when the child is ready to self-manage and needs staff only to supervise. The school or setting policy should include details of whether children may carry and administer their own medicines. The safety of other children needs to be considered in this policy, and it is advisable to gain written parental consent and advice from the prescriber. Where children are self-administering CDs, these should always be kept locked away in safe custody.

Record keeping

Keeping records is proof that agreed procedures have been carried out and offers protection to staff who have responsibility for medicines administration. It is a regulatory requirement that written records of medicines administered to children must be kept in all early years settings (DfES, 2005). Parents must then be asked to sign the record book to acknowledge the entry. There is no similar legal requirement for schools to keep records of medicines given to pupils; however, it is good practice to do so. As a minimum record, the name, date, dosage given, time given and the signature of the person administering the dose and a witness should be recorded.

Refusing to take medicines

If a child refuses to take some or all of the medicine, they should not be forced to do so. The refusal should be documented in the notes as well as the action taken. The procedure to take if a child refuses should be set out in the school or setting policy, or it may be included in a child's individual healthcare plan. Parents should be informed of the refusal on the same day. If the child's refusal could result in an emergency, the parent or a health professional should be informed immediately and emergency procedures followed.

Activity 5.4   *Communication*

You are a school nurse and have been contacted by telephone at lunchtime because 8-year-old Jonathon is refusing to take his medicine.

- What should you do?

An outline answer is provided at the end of the chapter.

The disposal of medicines

Parents should be responsible for the collection of all medicines at the end of term, and for the disposal of any out-of-date medicines by returning them to the pharmacy. Any medicines not collected by parents at the end of term should be returned to the local pharmacy for safe disposal. All needles and sharps must be disposed of into sharps boxes, which parents can obtain on prescription from their GP. The local authority environmental service is responsible for the collection and disposal of sharps boxes.

> ## Chapter summary
>
> This chapter has outlined the responsibilities of registered nurses and nurse managers for the safe storage of medicines. Good practice for the supply and ordering of medicines, including controlled drugs, both in the community and hospital settings has been described, and the chapter has covered procedures for the safe storage of vaccines, including transportation, the disposal and return of medicines, and the management of cytotoxic drugs, including spillage and waste disposal. The chapter ended with a description of good practice in the storage and administration of medicines in schools and other settings.

Activities: brief outline answers

Activity 5.1 CD cupboard keys (page 120)

You should not hand the keys over to the doctor. You should go with him to the CD cupboard and check out the drug with him, entering the details and signing against the stock balance in the CD record book. You should also check the patient prescription and accompany the doctor to the patient to witness the correct administration.

Activity 5.2 Vaccine refrigeration (page 124)

The first action you should take is to correct the situation by reinserting the plug and turning the power to the fridge back on. You then need to note and record the current temperature of the fridge. You should not immediately throw out the affected vaccines. Mark the vaccines that are in the fridge so that they are easily identifiable, and do not use them until the vaccines' effectiveness is determined. You must ensure that the fridge is working properly and, if not, move the vaccines to one that is. You then need to call the immunisation service with the following information that will be stored in the minimum–maximum thermometer.

- The current temperature of the fridge and the minimum and maximum temperature reached.
- The amount of time the temperature was outside the normal vaccine storage range.
- Whether the vaccine has been previously exposed to temperatures below the storage range.

The immunisation service will inform you of the feasibility of the vaccines or whether they need to be returned to the pharmacy for destruction. An incident form must always be completed to ensure that any necessary actions are taken to avoid further occurrences.

You may need to access some vaccines from another community clinic to carry out your clinic and you can replace these later.

Activity 5.3 Morphine discrepancy (page 126)

Any discrepancy in the total number of medicines must immediately be reported to the care manager. The care manager must immediately investigate the loss or discrepancy. First, you must double-check your count, ensuring that you have not missed any medication that is still inside the packaging. Check with the parents or carers to establish if they can offer any further information or explanation. You must record the incident in Amy's records and on the medication chart, including the date, time and your signature. The nurses who have been visiting Amy previously must be contacted to check for any drug discrepancies during the last visit. Amy's GP should be contacted to check if the doctors have administered or removed any CDs from Amy's home. Again, this action must be recorded in Amy's notes. The community pharmacist must be contacted to check the delivery of any CDs to the patient's house. An incident form must be completed and forwarded to the Risk Management Department as soon as possible. The care manager must report the incident to the appropriate senior managers and the police must be informed if there is reason to suspect theft of the drug.

Activity 5.4 Refusal to take medicine (page 129)

First, you need to establish if the medicine that Jonathon is refusing could potentially lead to a medical emergency (e.g. insulin) and if necessary emergency procedures should be carried out, such as calling for an ambulance. If there is no potential emergency, you should advise the designated member of staff to contact Jonathon's parents to inform them of his refusal and discuss further options. If necessary, a parent may be required to come to the school to administer the medication themselves.

Further reading

Department of Health (DH) (2007) *Safer Management of Controlled Drugs: A guide to good practice in secondary care (England)*. London: Department of Health.

This provides useful guidance for good practice for those who are involved in the day-to-day management of CDs in secondary care and for those who are responsible for making sure that CDs are managed safely in their organisations. It is available on the department's website at **www.dh.gov.uk**.

National Prescribing Centre (NPC) (2009) *A Guide to Good Practice in the Management of CDs in Primary Care (England)*, 3rd edition. Liverpool: NPC.

This is a useful practice guide on record keeping and is available online at **www.npci.org.uk/cd/ public/docs/controlled_drugs_third_edition.pdf**.

Useful websites

www.anaphylaxis.org.uk

The Anaphylaxis Campaign is a UK charity that aims to meet the needs of the growing numbers of people at risk from severe allergic reactions (anaphylaxis) by providing information and support relating to foods and other triggers, such as latex, drugs and insect stings.

www.asthma.org.uk

Asthma UK (formerly the National Asthma Campaign) provides information to help develop effective policies for dealing with asthma in schools and childcare settings.

www.dh.gov.uk

Current and past Department of Health publications, including statistical reports, surveys, press releases, circulars and legislation, are available in electronic format from this website.

www.epilepsysociety.org.uk

The National Society for Epilepsy is a medical charity working for everyone affected by epilepsy, through research, awareness campaigns and expert care.

www.ncb.org.uk/cdc

The Council for Disabled Children works to influence national policy that impacts upon disabled children and children with special educational needs (SEN) and their families.

Chapter 6
Medicines administration in children's nursing

> ## NMC Standards for Pre-registration Nursing Education
>
> This chapter will address the following competencies:
>
> ### Domain 3: Nursing practice and decision making
>
> *Generic standard for competence:*
>
> All nurses must practise autonomously, compassionately, skilfully and safely, and must maintain dignity and promote health and wellbeing. They must assess and meet the full range of essential physical and mental health needs of people of all ages who come into their care. Where necessary they must be able to provide safe and effective immediate care to all people prior to accessing or referring to specialist services irrespective of their field of practice. All nurses must also meet more complex and coexisting needs for people in their own nursing field of practice, in any setting including hospital, community and at home. All practice should be informed by the best available evidence and comply with local and national guidelines. Decision-making must be shared with service users, carers and families and informed by critical analysis of a full range of possible interventions, including the use of up-to-date technology. All nurses must also understand how behaviour, culture, socioeconomic and other factors, in the care environment and its location, can affect health, illness, health outcomes and public health priorities and take this into account in planning and delivering care.
>
> *Field standard for competence:*
>
> **Children's nurses** must be able to care safely and effectively for children and young people in all settings, and recognise their responsibility for safeguarding them. They must be able to deliver care to meet essential and complex physical and mental health needs informed by deep understanding of biological, psychological and social factors throughout infancy, childhood and adolescence.
>
> *Competencies:*
>
> 6. All nurses must practise safely by being aware of the correct use, limitations and hazards of common interventions, including nursing activities, treatments, the calculation and administration of medicines, and the use of medical devices and equipment. The nurse must be able to evaluate their use, report any concerns promptly through appropriate channels and modify care where necessary to maintain safety. They must contribute to the collection of local and national data and formulation of policy on risks, hazards and adverse outcomes.
>
> *continued opposite . . .*

continued . . . .

6.1 **Children's nurses** must have numeracy skills for medicines management, assessment, measuring, monitoring and recording which recognise the particular vulnerability of infants and young children in relation to accurate medicines calculation.

NMC Essential Skills Clusters

This chapter will address the following ESCs:

Cluster: Medicines management

38. People can trust the newly registered graduate nurse to administer medicines safely and in a timely manner, including controlled drugs.

39. People can trust a newly registered graduate nurse to keep and maintain accurate records using information technology, where appropriate, within a multi-disciplinary framework as a leader and as part of a team and in a variety of care settings including at home.

Chapter aims

By the end of this chapter, you should be able to:

* use a prescription chart correctly and maintain accurate records;
* safely and effectively prepare and administer medicines via different routes;
* recognise anaphylaxis and manage the condition;
* report contraindications, side effects and adverse reactions.

Case study

As a sister on a paediatric surgical ward, I was asked by a staff nurse to second-check some medication that she was administering. The ward was extremely busy, and a parent had asked the staff nurse if she could give her child some paracetamol suspension, as the child had returned from theatre and was in pain. The staff nurse went to the medicines cupboard and prepared the medication without me because she could see I was busy. The staff nurse locked the medicines cupboard and brought me the medicine pot with the 10mL of 'paracetamol suspension' for me to check against the prescription chart. I questioned the staff nurse as the colour of the liquid was clear and did not look like paracetamol suspension. The staff nurse immediately realised her error; she had not been concentrating and had measured out 10mL of trimeprazine tartrate, a drug that we frequently administered as a pre-anaesthetic medication.

continued overleaf . . .

continued . . . .

This is an example of a near-miss drug error. If the wrong drug had been administered, both the staff nurse and I would have been accountable. Procedure for both nurses checking the medicine bottle and the dose was not followed and this had contributed to the error. The staff nurse had felt she was capable of preparing a simple dose of paracetamol without the need for a colleague to check on her. When under pressure, it is tempting to cut corners in order to get the job done. It is impossible to know how many similar drug errors or dosing errors go undetected every day. In order to prevent such errors there are strict guidelines and procedures to follow when preparing and administering medication.

Introduction

The procedure for the safe administration of medicines will be discussed in this chapter. You will be introduced to a typical prescription chart and how to use one in order to administer medicines and maintain accurate records. There are many different routes of medicines administration, with which you must be familiar. The most common include the oral, enteral, intravenous, intramuscular, subcutaneous, rectal, buccal, ocular, aural, transdermal, inhalation and nasal routes. This chapter includes the procedure for the safe preparation and administration of medicine via each of these routes. Any nurse who administers medication should be trained to identify adverse reactions and report errors. The chapter will include this, along with how to recognise anaphylaxis and manage the condition.

Administering medication

As a registered nurse remember that you are accountable for your actions and omissions. Every time you administer any medication you must use your professional judgement, knowledge and skills. You must ensure that the drug is legally prescribed by an authorised health professional and, wherever possible, that the child/parent's informed consent was obtained and they are aware of the treatment.

Cautions, contraindications and interactions

Before administering a drug dose you need to check there are no contraindications to administration because of the child's age or clinical condition. Many drugs are contraindicated in certain conditions, in particular pregnancy, renal and liver disease. You must be aware of your patient's clinical condition and check in the relevant section of the BNFC. Some medicines must only be administered with caution in certain conditions or patient groups and this will be indicated in the BNFC. For example, some topical medicines should be used with caution on broken or inflamed skin. Many drugs should be used with caution in pregnancy or while breastfeeding. Two or more medicines given to the same patient at the same time may interact with each other. It is possible for one drug to cause an increase or a decrease in the effectiveness of the other. Sometimes there will be some other adverse reaction. Before administering more than one medication to a child you should check in the appendix of the BNFC for interactions. The following activity is to highlight the importance of checking in the BNFC the licensed use, indications, dose side effects and the contraindications before administering a medicine.

Activity 6.1   *Evidence-based practice and research*

Three-year-old Charlotte was admitted to the ward three days ago with diarrhoea and vomiting, from which she is recovering well. Her mother has asked the doctor if Charlotte could have some treatment for the red itchy rash she has between her toes. The doctor has diagnosed this as athlete's foot (tinea pedis) and prescribes salicylic acid paint twice daily. Charlotte is not prescribed any other medications, and she has no other medical conditions and no allergies.

- You are the first nurse to administer the paint. Is there any reason why you should not do so?

An outline answer is provided at the end of the chapter.

Administering a drug dose

Check that the prescription is current and complete, and that it does not conflict with any other charts in use. The hospital prescription must be legible and indelible, and must include:

- the child's full name and hospital number;
- the child's age and date of birth;
- the child's weight in kilograms (is the weight reasonable for the child's age?);
- the hospital and ward.

Before administration can take place, the following items must be present as part of the actual prescription:

- date;
- medicine (generic name written in full or brand name if appropriate);
- dose (never accept unapproved abbreviations, e.g. µg);
- medicine form and strength (e.g. paracetamol 500mg tablets or paracetamol suspension 120mg/5mL);
- frequency of administration or time for administration;
- route (i.e. oral, nasogastric, rectal, intravenous etc.);
- start and finish dates;
- prescriber's signature in full for each medicine prescribed.

If any of the above information is missing or unclear, do not administer the drug; refer back to the prescriber to amend the prescription.

Only administer drugs against a doctor's verbal order in an absolute emergency and ensure that it is followed up in writing as soon as possible. Write it down and repeat it back to ensure accuracy.

Activity 6.2 — *Reflection*

Try to think of a situation you have been in where yourself or a senior colleague might have been asked to administer a drug on the verbal order of a prescriber.

- What were the circumstances?
- Did you administer the drug?
- What do you consider to be an absolute emergency in relation to drug administration?

Outline answers are provided at the end of the chapter.

Figure 6.1 is an example of a typical hospital patient medicines administration or prescription chart, or what is sometimes known as a patient specific direction (PSD). Note the different sections for regular medication, once-only medication or pre-anaesthetic medication and infusion therapy. You must ensure that all boxes are completed on the correct part of the prescription chart.

DRUG SENSITIVITY (must be completed in RED ink)		Hosp no:	D.O.B.
Weight (Kg):	Height (M):	Surname: **LABEL**	
Consultant:	Ward:	First Name(s):	
Sheet No.		Address:	Sex: M/F

DRUGS OMITTED
R   Refused
U   Drug unavailable
O   Omitted-medical instruction
I   Instructions illegible or unclear
V   Patient vomiting
D   Drowsy or asleep
A   Absent from ward
X   Other reason, specify on chart

PRESCRIBER
Use approved names legibly, BLOCK LETTERS
Metric doses and English instructions
Sign legibly
Drug sensitivity box must be rewritten NOT altered
Only one chart to be used at any time
Discontinue a drug by drawing a line through it and subsequent record boxes. Fill in 'Finish Date' or 'Cancel' box

ONCE-ONLY MEDICATION AND PRE-ANAESTHETIC MEDICATION

DATE	DRUG (APPROVED NAME)	ROUTE	DOSE	TIME	SIGNATURE	GIVEN BY	TIME	PHARM.

INFUSION THERAPY

DATE	FLUID	VOL.	RATE	BATCH NO.	DRUG ADDED	DOSE	DR's SIGNATURE	TIME BEGUN	ENDED

Figure 6.1: A patient medicines administration chart

REGULAR PRESCRIPTIONS	Patient's Name:												Hosp. No.:								

YEAR:	MONTH:		DATE →																		
			TIME ↓		Week 1						Week 2						Week 3				
DRUG (approved name)			0600																		
DOSE	**ROUTE**	**Pharmacy**	0800																		
Instructions/Duration			1300																		
Start Date & Time		Init. Cont.	1800																		
Signature			2200																		
CANCEL (Date & Sig.)			0000																		

DRUG (approved name)			0600																		
DOSE	ROUTE	Pharmacy	0800																		
Instructions/Duration			1300																		
Start Date & Time		Init. Cont.	1800																		
Signature			2200																		
CANCEL (Date & Sig.)			0000																		

DRUG (approved name)			0600																		
DOSE	ROUTE	Pharmacy	0800																		
Instructions/Duration			1300																		
Start Date & Time		Init. Cont.	1800																		
Signature			2200																		
CANCEL (Date & Sig.)			0000																		

DRUG (approved name)			0600																		
DOSE	ROUTE	Pharmacy	0800																		
Instructions/Duration			1300																		
Start Date & Time		Init. Cont.	1800																		
Signature			2200																		
CANCEL (Date & Sig.)			0000																		

Figure 6.1: Continued

The following activity should help you with the interpretation of a PSD.

Activity 6.3 — Critical thinking

Read the following PSD and answer the questions.

ONCE-ONLY MEDICATION AND PRE-ANAESTHETIC MEDICATION								
DATE	DRUG (APPROVED NAME)	ROUTE	DOSE	TIME	SIGNATURE	GIVEN	TIME BY	PHARM.
20/10/ 2010	Vallergan	PO	30mg	1–2 hrs pre-op	*K Jones*	*RJ*	0800	*TC*

- What date and time was the drug to be given?
- What is wrong with the drug name as it is written?

Answers are provided at the end of the chapter.

You should now be familiar with a typical patient's medicines administration chart or PSD, and how to interpret the information. The following section will explain what information you must have available and what you must do before administering a medicine.

Before administration

Two practitioners should check and administer medicines unless single-nurse administration has been specified in local policy. First, you must both check that the medicine has not already been given by checking the signature space in the patient administration chart, as well as other charts such as anaesthetic charts or separate intravenous and oral charts. Ensure only one patient medicines administration chart is in use and that it is clear.

You must check that the child is not allergic or intolerant to the prescribed drug by checking the chart and with the parent. Ensure that there are no therapeutic duplications, for example paracetamol and co-codamol (containing paracetamol) have not been prescribed concurrently. Use the BNFC to check that the dose is appropriate and that it is not contraindicated for that particular child. Make yourself aware of the drug indications, interactions and side effects.

Both practitioners will now need to independently calculate the amount of medicine to be administered before comparing answers. If you are unsure of the correct answer you may need to involve a third person. Next, prepare your medicine after washing your hands. Double-check the label on the medicine container against the prescription and be aware of medicines with similar names (for example salbutamol and salmeterol). Check that the medicine has not expired and that storage instructions have been adhered to (for example, some drugs **denature** if not kept in the fridge). The checking practitioner should witness the preparation and measurement of the medicine and agree that the correct volume has been prepared.

Once prepared, the medicine should never be left unlabelled or unattended. Before administering it, you must check the patient administration chart against the child's identity bracelet and verify the name, hospital number and date of birth.

The following activity should help you with the interpretation of a PSD.

Activity 6.4   **Critical thinking**

Read the following patient specific direction and answer the questions.

REGULAR PRESCRIPTIONS	Name: Scarlett Moss					Hosp. No.: 6889345		
YEAR: 2010								
MONTH: April								
DATE ⟶	3rd	4th	5th	6th	7th			
TIME ▼	Week 1					Week 2		Week 3
DRUG (approved name) Amoxicillin	0600	R B	R B	R B				
DOSE 125mg ROUTE PO Pharmacy TC	1200							
Instructions/ Duration 8-hourly	1400	T C	V T C	I W	I W			
Start date Init. Cont. & time 5 days 3/4/10 1800	1800							
Signature L. Gilbert	2200	R B	R B	R B				
CANCEL (Date & Sig.) 8/4/10 K. Summers	2400							

• What is the route of administration?
• What date and time will the last dose be administered?
• What does the 'V' stand for at 1400hrs on 5th April?

Answers are provided at the end of the chapter.

The following section explains what you must do during and after the administration of a medicine.

During administration

You must always be aware of and follow local policy for medicines administration. Students must always be under direct supervision of a qualified nurse and never administer medicines alone. Medical staff must also have medicines checked by a second person when possible. When you are confident you have completed all the necessary pre-administration checks and have checked the child's wristband against the patient administration chart, you may administer the medicine. Always remain with the child until the full dose has been taken. Do not leave medicines on bedside lockers as this endangers other children on the ward and you cannot be sure the medicine will be taken on time. If the medicine is being administered by intravenous infusion, ensure that the infusion is completed on time.

Parents administering medication to their child

Parents must be supervised when administering medicines to their own children, unless an agreement has been made with the senior nurse. In some circumstances it may be appropriate for the child to self-administer their own medicine. The patient medicines administration chart should document medicines administered by parents or child.

Record keeping

You should always sign the patient medicines administration chart as soon as the medicine has been administered to avoid a duplicate dose being given. If a medicine was not administered, you must record the reason why and inform the prescriber. Omission of medicines can have serious consequences in some circumstances, so you should record your reasons why. Ensure that any medicines given by parents or self-administered are recorded.

Case study

In a GP surgery I once worked in, a busy GP was asked by a patient to administer their regular Depo-Provera contraceptive injection. The GP went to the fridge where the medication was usually stored and took out the injection. Without double-checking, the GP administered it to the patient. After the patient left the room the GP realised while writing the notes that the injection given was actually a depot antipsychotic medication, Depixol. The consequences for the patient were serious.

This story may sound unlikely and extreme, but it is actually true. The patient had to be recalled and the error explained and rectified. The circumstances that contributed to this error were as follows.

- The GP did not normally administer the contraceptive injection; it was usually the practice nurse's role.
- The GP was stressed and had very limited time.
- The injections had similar names and were stored next to each other in the fridge.
- The GP had no second-checker or prescription chart to refer to.

Some hospitals now store medicines according to frequency of use, rather than alphabetically, which saves time and reduces mistakes of this sort.

Concept summary: Six rights of medication administration

As the person administering a drug, you have the last opportunity to identify an error before a patient is harmed. Always recheck the following 'six Rs' rigorously even though you are busy and they have been checked previously:

- right drug
- right dose
- right route
- right time
- right patient
- right documentation completed.

Routes and methods of administration

This section describes the methods of administration for the different routes most commonly used. The route of administration will have been decided by the prescriber based on the patient's medical condition and medicines available. The route of administration should be clearly indicated on the patient medicines administration chart.

Oral administration

The oral route (by mouth) is the most common form of drug administration in children. Medicines for oral administration are supplied in many forms and include liquids (suspensions, elixirs or syrups), tablets, capsules, granules and powders. Oral medicines are available in a number of different strengths and flavours (e.g. paracetamol 120mg/5mL and 240mg/5mL).

Tablets and capsules

Tablets are easier to store and transport and do not contain sugar, so when possible should be the form of choice. Children under the age of about 4 years may have difficulty swallowing tablets and capsules, and may be at risk of choking or aspiration. Tablets and capsules can be supplied as enteric coated and sustained release for better absorption. These tablets should never be crushed or the capsules opened. If a tablet or capsule is the only oral form available of the drug, check with the pharmacist if it is safe to crush or open the capsule. It can then be mixed with a small amount (no more than a tablespoon) of sterile water or pleasant-tasting liquid or food. Medicines should never be mixed with the child's milk or essential foods as the child may then associate these foods with a bitter taste and refuse to eat them. Medicines supplied as powders, granules or sprinkles should only be mixed with a small quantity of food or drink (teaspoonful) to ensure that the whole amount is taken. Never mix into the whole feed or a bowlful, as the child may not complete the full amount. Remember also, some medicines are absorbed more completely without food.

Swallowing tablets

The age at which children learn to swallow tablets varies, as do other areas of development, as it requires a certain amount of coordination. It is worth encouraging children to learn to swallow tablets as they can be less unpleasant than liquids. Older children should be encouraged to fully participate in the administration of medicines and to self-administer. This is particularly important in children with long-term conditions such as cystic fibrosis, who require large and frequent doses of medication. When instructing younger children on how to swallow tablets, you should encourage them to place the tablet or capsule towards the back of their tongue before swallowing with water. It may help to drink through a straw, as this may distract them from concentrating on the tablet.

Liquid medicines

Liquid medicine preparations are more appropriate for infants and younger children as they are easier to swallow. Liquid medicines consist of a given weight of drug dissolved or suspended in a given volume of liquid. Manufacturers often try to mask the bitter tastes of medicines with sugars to make them more palatable and attractive to young children. These preparations often contain glucose, fructose and sucrose, and can contribute to dental caries in children, particularly with frequent doses over long periods. You should therefore, when possible, always request a sugar-free formulation, and encourage prescribers to add 'SF' (sugar-free) to their prescriptions.

Liquid medications, when settled, may be more concentrated at the bottom of the bottle, so always shake the bottle before administration to ensure even drug distribution. You must use a calibrated medicine spoon, cup, plastic syringe or dropper to measure the correct dose for administration. For most medicines, it is acceptable to measure doses in multiples of 5mL on a medicine spoon or in a measuring cup (see Figures 6.2 and 6.3). You must use an oral syringe without a needle (never a parenteral syringe) to measure amounts less than 5mL accurately. Some medicines come supplied with a dropper to measure a specific dose.

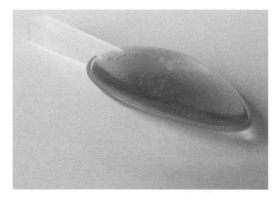

Figure 6.2: A medicine spoon

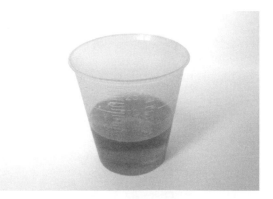

Figure 6.3: A measuring cup

Medicine pipettes

Some medicines such as Nystan oral suspension and Lanoxin elixir are supplied with a graduated pipette, which should be used for the measurement of all doses. The pipette has a soft bulb to suck up and squeeze out medicine and makes accurate dosing to young babies by mouth easier (see Figure 6.4). Parents should be instructed on how to use the pipette to measure the correct dose.

Oral syringes

An oral syringe (see Figure 6.5) can be used for accurately measuring small doses of liquid medicine to be administered to children by mouth. They are available in different sizes, most commonly 1mL, 2.5mL and 5mL, but are also available in 10mL and larger sizes.

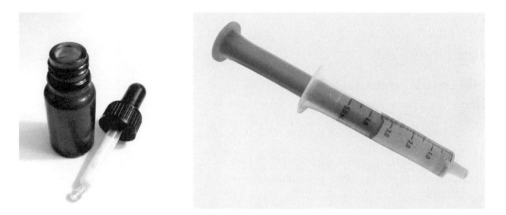

Figure 6.4: A medicine pipette   *Figure 6.5: An oral syringe*

Administering liquid medicine

Ask the parent or carer to hold the infant comfortably on their lap and ensure the child is held upright or semi-upright to avoid aspiration. When using a dropper or oral syringe, you should direct the liquid to the side of the mouth towards the back (see Figure 6.6). Administer the medicine slowly, a half mL at a time, allowing the child to swallow each time. Infants may be given medicine via a teat without the bottle attached. Place the medication directly into the teat and allow the infant to suck without allowing any air into the teat. If a child is old enough, allow them to take the medicine from a medicine spoon or cup, or the child may enjoy squirting the medicine from a syringe into their own mouth. Remember to use positive reinforcement of praise and to encourage participation through play.

Never force medicines into a child's mouth or hold the child's nose. This risks aspiration and will lose a child's trust as it is unpleasant. Advise parents against using household spoons to measure doses, as they are not calibrated and will deliver an incorrect dose of medication.

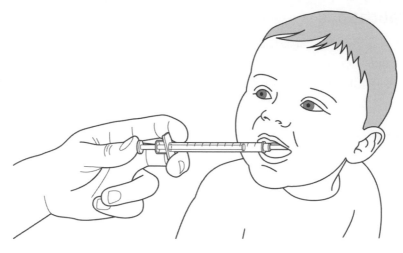

Figure 6.6: Giving a baby medicine from an oral syringe

Administration via enteral tubes

Drugs are frequently administered to children via feeding tubes. Oral medications may be administered via nasogastric, orogastric, gastrostomy, naso-jejunal and jejunostomy tubes, if the child is unable to take the medicine orally. The medicine must be prescribed via the specific enteral route rather than orally (i.e. the drug chart should specify 'via gastrostomy' or 'via jejunostomy'). The tube allows the medication to be placed directly into the stomach or jejunal area. Medicines that are absorbed in the stomach should not be given via jejunal tubes as the stomach is bypassed, so you must check that the drug is absorbed from the site of delivery.

To administer medication this way it needs to be in liquid form. Avoid crushed tablet or opened capsules when possible as tablet fragments may block tubing. If unavoidable, crush to a fine powder and disperse completely with water. Thick liquids may block fine-bore tubes and may be unsuitable or need to be diluted further. Injection solutions may be suitable for administering via enteral tubes.

Medicines that should not be crushed

You should only crush tablets and open capsules as a last resort after checking that this is safe with a pharmacist and that a liquid preparation is not available.

- Enteric coated (EC) tablets are designed with a coating that resists gastric acid to protect the drug and reduce gastric side effects.
- Modified release (MR), slow/sustained release (SR), long acting (LA) and extended release (XL, XR) tablets are specifically designed to release the drug over a long period of time. Crushing these will cause the entire drug to be released at once and will cause toxic side effects.
- Cytotoxic preparations and hormones should not be crushed for administration due to the risk of exposure to staff from the powdered drug.
- **Lipid-based** drugs such as phenytoin can adhere to the side of the tube and cause incomplete dose delivery.

Legal implications

Crushing tablets, opening capsules and administrating drugs via feeding tubes usually falls outside a drug's product licence. This will mean that the prescriber of the drug and the practitioner administering the drug must accept liability for any adverse effects that result from this method of administration.

Drug interactions

If the absorption of a drug is affected by food or antacids, it is likely to be affected by enteral feeds. Some interactions can be clinically significant so, wherever possible, give drugs during a break in the enteral feed.

Clinically significant interactions

The absorption of phenytoin, **carbamazapine** and **digoxin** can be affected by enteral feeds and the child's blood plasma levels should be checked regularly. It may be necessary to increase the dose of these drugs when they are administered via feeding tubes. Anticipate the need for dose reduction when enteral feeding is discontinued. Phenytoin suspension can also stick to the side of the feeding tube and prevent administration of the full dose. Antacids can also bind to the protein in an enteral feed and block the tube. Enteral feeds may reduce significantly the absorption of penicillins, tetracyclines, rifampicin and ciprofloxacin and higher doses may be needed.

Enteral tube administration

Wash your hands and wear gloves. Use an oral, enteral or catheter-tipped syringe to administer the drug and, if necessary, a specially designed connector to attach to the tube. Use an appropriately sized syringe for the drug volume, and take care not to apply too much pressure so as to split the tube (check the manufacturer's guidelines). Remember, never use syringes intended for intravenous use as there is a risk of accidental intravenous administration. You must always check for correct placement of the tube before administration, and tubes should be flushed with water (sterile water for neonates) before and after drug administration. Enteral feeds should be stopped before the medicine is given and flushed through with a small amount of water. Do not add medication directly to an enteral feeding formula; each drug should be administered separately through an appropriate access site, flushing between each drug with an appropriate volume of water. You must utilise a flush volume that is appropriate to the size of the child and the size of the tube (15mL of water would be an appropriate adult volume, whereas in neonates the volume of flush must be carefully limited to avoid overloading with fluids). Never mix medications together due to the risk of drug incompatibility. The enteral feed may need to be interrupted for short periods of 30 minutes or longer before and after administration, when appropriate, to avoid altering the bioavailability of the drug. Always restart feeding in a timely manner to avoid compromising the child's nutritional status.

> ## Case studies
>
> *The following case studies are from a National Patient Safety Agency (NPSA) Safety Alert (2007).*
>
> *'Child received phenytoin oral suspension by incorrect route – was administered via a Hickman line (intravenously) instead of the gastrostomy tube (enterally).' Outcome no harm.*
>
> *'Patient given enteral (gastric) feed down Hickman line (intravenously) in error. Patient had severe back pain, reduced oxygen concentration in blood, increased pulse as fat embolus entered subclavian vein leading to the heart and lungs.' Outcome severe harm.*

The above case studies emphasise the importance of never using intravenous syringes to measure and administer oral liquids, as they can inadvertently be administered by the wrong route.

Clearing blockages

The most common causes of feeding tube blockage are inadequate flushing and medication administration. Blockage of feeding tubes is a serious problem that can deprive a child of essential drugs, fluids and nutrients, and cause unnecessary tube replacement. You should try to prevent this with adequate flushing and correct dilution of medicines. To clear blockages, an attempt should be made to aspirate to remove particles and this should be followed by an attempt to flush through with warm water. You should never apply excessive pressure due to risk of the tube splitting. It is possible that sugar-free carbonated drinks may be slightly better than water at clearing blocked feeding tubes. However, mildly acidic liquids such as Coca-Cola and pineapple juice can coagulate protein in feeds and cause further blockage (BMA et al., 2010). If these measures fail, seek expert advice. The family should be given a point of contact for advice if this happens.

Intravenous administration

The intravenous (IV) route involves the administration of medicine directly into a vein. Compared with other routes of administration, the IV route is the fastest way to deliver medications to the body. Some medications can only be given intravenously and it is the preferred route of administration if the child is critically ill. Medicines may be given as a bolus injection or continuous and intermittent infusions. Peripheral or central access devices can be used, as appropriate to the circumstances of the child and the pharmacological properties of the medicine. As a registered nurse you must be trained and demonstrate competence in order to administer IV drugs and drug infusions. Risks in administering drugs via the IV route include infection, **extravasation**, **infiltration** and **phlebitis**. There is also a higher risk of anaphylaxis with this route.

IV medication is ideally given in an environment where emergency resuscitation equipment is available. Adrenaline should always be readily available because of the risk of anaphylaxis. Community nurses should carry adrenaline when administering IV drugs and be appropriately trained to administer it without a prescription or medical supervision if needed in an emergency.

All registered nurses can check IV medications according to local policy, but they are prohibited from administering them unless they have received additional IV administration training. It is recommended that two registered nurses check the administration of IV medicines, although this is not practical for community nurses. The registered nurse must only administer those drugs with which they are familiar and of which they have an understanding of their actions. Student nurses should never attach or administer IV medicines to patients. To prepare IV medicines hands should be washed, gloves worn and a non-touch technique used. Surface contaminates should be cleaned from ampoules and vials with alcohol swabs. Filter needles are recommended to draw up medications from glass ampoules and vials to reduce the risk of glass particle contamination. Ensure a sharps box is readily available for disposal of needles, which should never be resheathed or detached from the syringe.

Peripheral IV therapy sites

Medicines are administered via peripheral IV sites if the child is unable to take the medicine orally due to vomiting or an inability to swallow, or because the medicine is not absorbed via the gastrointestinal route. The peripheral route may also be used in an emergency when an immediate effect is needed, or may be preferred if the child is critically ill. A cannula can be sited and remain *in situ* for 72 hours before resiting, therefore necessitating fewer injections.

Common sites for peripheral IV therapy include the hands, forearms and feet. In infants under 1 year, scalp veins are sometimes used if access is difficult elsewhere. Scalp veins are easy to visualise due to only a thin covering of subcutaneous tissue. Shaving the head is often necessary and this can be distressing for parents. Peripheral IV sites need to be checked before each medicine administration and hourly if a continuous intravenous infusion (IVI) is in progress. Signs of phlebitis or infection include redness, swelling or pain around the IV site or along the path of the cannula. If this occurs it should be reported to medical staff and documented, and the cannula should be removed and resited.

Central IV therapy

In central IV therapy, medication is delivered through a large vein such as the vena cava or jugular, subclavian or femoral veins. The device is inserted surgically and is usually used when the child has limited peripheral access and requires IV fluid or medication over longer periods. Devices include central lines (Hickman/Broviac/Groshong), implantable ports (Port-a-Cath/Mediport) and peripheral inserted central catheters (PICCs). They are an advantage because they can avoid multiple IV attempts and reduce painful procedures and fear. The risks include thrombosis due to partial occlusion of the vessel, local infection at the site and, more seriously, septicaemia due to direct access to the central circulation.

Administration via central catheters

Some catheters have double or triple lumen (spaces in the middle of the tube), allowing different treatments to be given at the same time. Each lumen will have a separate cap to which a syringe or infusion can be attached. Air must not be allowed to get into the line and clamps must be applied or caps in place when not in use.

Monitoring for complications

Infection can develop locally where a central line is inserted, and signs include redness, swelling or oozing. If the child develops a temperature antiobiotics will be required, or removal of the line. Signs of a thrombosis (blood clot) around a line include redness, swelling or tenderness in the arm, chest area or up into the neck. Report any shortness of breath or tightness in the chest to doctors immediately.

Intramuscular administration

The intramuscular route involves the administration of medicine directly into a muscle. Due to the discomfort of this route it is rarely used in children. It is used when other routes are not possible or do not allow effective absorption of the medication. This route is used for the administration of vaccines and may be preferable for a single dose of medication to resiting an IV cannula. The choice of site should take into consideration the child's age and physical state, and the volume of drug to be given. You should choose a site free from skin lesions, inflammation or infection. Intramuscular injection should be avoided in children with bleeding disorders.

The needle to give the medication is selected according to the size of the child and muscle depth. The needle should be long enough to reach muscle but not hit the bone. Choosing the correct needle length in order to deliver the drug to the muscle layer reduces complications such as pain, bruising and abscess formation (Cook and Murtagh, 2005; Zaybak et al., 2007). The use of a 25mm (blue) has been shown to reduce local reactions from vaccines (Diggle and Deeks, 2000; Diggle et al., 2006). A 25mm (23-gauge blue) or 25mm (25-gauge orange) needle is recommended for intramuscular injections in infants, children and adults (DH, 2006). Only in very small or preterm infants is a 16mm needle suitable for intramuscular injection. A longer length 38mm needle may be required in a young person of adult size and individual assessment should be made (Poland et al., 1997; Zuckerman, 2000).

Maximum recommended injection volumes are poorly researched and are unclear. In an adult, in a large muscle, the maximum volume recommended is 4–5mL and, in a smaller muscle, 1–2mL (Workman, 1999). These volumes should be reduced for children and less than 1mL is recommended for all sites in a child under 2 years (Hemsworth, 2000). At all times use your clinical judgement on the volume a child can tolerate, based on the muscle size and the viscosity of the medicine. There is some evidence that smaller injected volumes help absorption and are less likely to cause a reaction (John and Stevenson, 1995). The DH (2006) recommends dividing doses between two sites if the volume to be injected is greater than 3mL or 4mL.

Potential complications

There are several potential complications that can be caused by the administration of intramuscular medicines. Complications include pain, anaphylaxis, and sterile and septic abscess formation if large-volume injections are given. Another long-term complication is needle phobia, which can occur following a traumatic intramuscular injection experience.

Sites for injection

The sites recommended for intramuscular injection in children are the deltoid and anterolateral thigh muscles (RCPCH/RCN, 2002). Vastus lateralis (the lateral aspect of the thigh) is the most common site for injections in infants. Rectus femoris (the middle of the front of the thigh) is a painful site and is therefore not recommended, except for ease of access and self-administration. A randomised study (Cook and Murtagh, 2003) comparing the ventrogluteal site with antero-lateral thigh injections in children aged 18 months and 2, 4 and 6 years found better parental acceptance and fewer adverse events in the ventrogluteal site (halfway between the hip and the head of the femur). Deltoid muscle (the lateral aspect of the upper arm) is commonly used for children over 5 years and for small-volume injections such as vaccines. It is not suitable for large volumes or repeated injections (RCPCH, 1999). The dorsogluteal site (the upper outer quadrant of the buttock) is not recommended for infants and young children due to the risk of sciatic nerve injury and poor absorption of vaccines (DH, 2006; RCPCH/RCN, 2002). Reduced absorption can occur, resulting in a sterile abscess if the injection is deposited into adipose tissue rather than muscle (Workman, 1999). The buttocks should only be used for large-volume injections such as immunoglobulin (RCPCH/RCN, 2002).

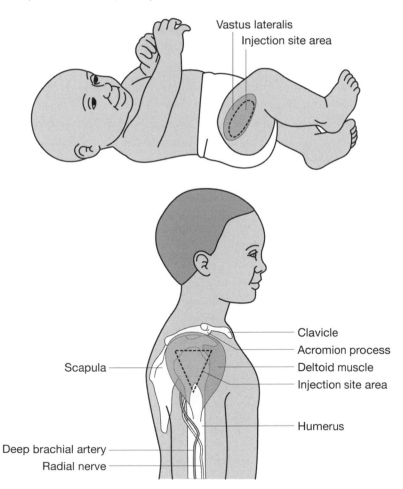

Figure 6.7: Suitable intramuscular injection sites

Intramuscular injection technique

This is the procedure to follow when you are giving a child an intramuscular injection.

First, prepare the medication using an appropriately sized syringe and discard the needle used to 'draw up' the solution and replace with a new needle to give the medication.

Intramuscular injections are less painful if the muscle is relaxed, and the child should be held securely by a parent or other adult to prevent movement. To relax the upper arm, the child should be sitting with the hand resting on the hip. Internal rotation of the femur helps to relax the gluteals in the buttocks. To achieve this, the child would need to be positioned prone on the bed with the knees apart and the toes pointing inwards. To relax the vastus lateralis, the knee should be slightly flexed.

Local anaesthetic can be considered, such as Ametop, EMLA, ice packs and ethyl chloride spray, but this will not relieve the deep muscle pain. Pressing on the skin for ten seconds before an injection can reduce the sensitivity of nerve endings and reduce pain.

Cleansing the skin before intramuscular injection is not routinely advised unless the child is immunocompromised or the skin is dirty (RCPCH/RCN, 2002). Gloves are not necessary, but some practitioners may prefer to wear non-sterile gloves to avoid the risk of contamination from blood or medicine.

The administration technique is as follows.

- Hold the skin around the site firmly with your free hand.
- The needle should be inserted at a 90-degree angle, deep enough to penetrate muscle but not touch bone.
- The skin should be stretched, not bunched, and it is not necessary to aspirate the syringe after the needle is introduced into the muscle (WHO, 2004).
- Inject the medication slowly at a rate no faster than 1mL per 10 seconds (Soanes, 2000).
- Allow 10 seconds before removal of the needle to allow the muscle fibres to absorb the solution.
- The needle should be removed slowly at a 90-degree angle.
- Release the retracted tissue to allow it to close over the needle track and prevent medication leaking out, and apply gentle pressure with a gauze swab or cotton-wool ball.
- Do not massage the site as this may cause local irritation. Gently exercising the limb afterwards may assist in absorption of the solution.

Post-injection

After you have given the child an injection, you should document the site used and the medicine given, and inspect the site after a few hours for adverse reactions. Inform the child or parent to report to you any excess pain, swelling or redness at the injection site.

The following activity is to check your understanding of intramuscular injection sites.

Activity 6.5   *Evidence-based practice and research*

James Dickson is a healthy 9 year old admitted to the accident and emergency department as he has fallen and fractured his right radius. He is in a lot of pain for which he has been prescribed intramuscular morphine sulphate.

•   What site would you choose to administer the injection?

An outline answer is provided at the end of the chapter.

Subcutaneous administration

The subcutaneous route is the administration of medication into the tissue just below the skin. The subcutaneous route is commonly used in paediatrics for a wide range of treatments, either by infusion or injection. Medicines given via the subcutaneous route include insulin, opioids and hormone treatments. Absorption of medication from the subcutaneous route is slower than from the intramuscular route, and the rate of absorption varies depending on the site used. Potential injection sites include the abdomen, buttocks, hips, lateral aspects of the thigh and the upper outer arms. This route is most frequently used for the administration of insulin in children with diabetes mellitus. As it is important that the insulin is absorbed at the same rate every day; ideally, the same injection site should be used at the same time each day, for example upper arm in the morning.

Subcutaneous injection technique

The technique is similar to giving an intramuscular injection, except that you use a much shorter 25G 19mm or 27G 13mm needle in order to minimise discomfort when inserting the needle to the correct depth.

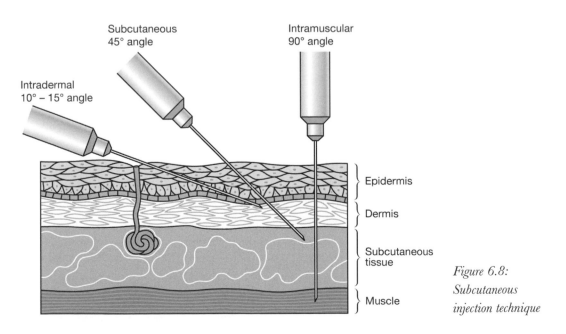

Figure 6.8: Subcutaneous injection technique

The administration technique is as follows.

- Give the injection at a 45-degree angle, avoiding the muscle by bunching the skin between your fingers.
- There is no need to aspirate the needle to check if a blood vessel has been punctured, as this is much less likely.
- Wash your hands and document in the same way as for other medication.

Rectal administration

Medication can be administered via the rectal route in the form of suppositories (paracetamol) and liquids (diazepam rectal tubes). The route is particularly useful when the intravenous route is difficult or oral medication cannot be tolerated due to nausea, vomiting or loss of consciousness. The rectal route is not as acceptable as other routes within some cultures as it is invasive. Rectal diazepam previously given for the management of convulsions has now been generally replaced with the use of buccal midazolam.

Rectal administration technique

This is the procedure to follow when giving a child medicine via the rectum.

- Wash your hands to prevent cross-infection.
- Explain the procedure to the child at a level that is appropriate to their understanding and ensure that informed consent is obtained.
- The child should be positioned comfortably on the left side with the right leg flexed.
- The tip of the suppository or enema can be moistened with water or a water-based lubricant (such as K-Y gel) before inserting.
- The rounded ended of the suppository is gently inserted into the anus and propelled forward.
- If possible, ask the child to 'hold on' to the suppository for five minutes.

Buccal administration

Buccal medications are administered to be absorbed rapidly into the bloodstream through the mucous membrane of the mouth. One commonly used in children is buccal midazolam for the management of status epilepticus. The route is more effective because it bypasses the digestive system, so swallowing the medication should be prevented. Buccal medications should not be administered if the mucous membranes are inflamed or have open sores.

Buccal administration technique

This is the procedure to follow when giving a child medicine via the buccal route.

- First, wash your hands and put on non-sterile gloves.
- Then open the child's mouth, and use an oral syringe to place the medication between the upper lip and gum of each side of the mouth.
- Ask the child to keep the medicine in the mouth for at least five minutes before swallowing.

Eye (ocular) administration

Medication can be administered directly to the eye in the form of drops or ointment.

Eye administration technique

This is the procedure to follow when giving a child medicine via the eye.

- Always wash your hands to prevent cross-infection.
- Shake the drops well to disperse the medication evenly.
- Eye drops should be labelled for individual patients and for right and left eye to prevent cross-infection.
- Explain the procedure to the child at a level that is appropriate to their understanding.
- Clean any sticky exudates around the eyelids first with gauze swabs and sterile water (you will need to wash your hands again).
- The child should be lying flat on the back or with head tilted back if seated in a chair.
- Ask the child to look up, while you gently pull the lower eyelid down and away from the eye.
- Gently administer the eye drop on to the conjunctiva behind the eyelid. Ointment should be gently applied in a fine strip 1–2cm long, taking care not to touch the eye with the end of the tube.
- Ask the child to close their eyes for one minute after instillation to avoid blinking, which would expel the medication into the nasolacrimal duct.
- If the child is prescribed more than one eye medication, administer drops before ointment, which can seal the eye and prevent absorption of the drops.
- You should wait five minutes between instilling drops and ointment into the same eye.
- Wash your hands and document in the same way as for other medication.

Ear (aural) administration

Medication can be administered directly to the ear in the form of drops or ointment.

Ear administration technique

This is the procedure to follow when giving a child medicine via the ear.

- Always wash your hands to prevent cross-infection.
- Shake the drops well to disperse the medication evenly.
- Explain the procedure to the child at a level that is appropriate to their understanding.
- The child should be lying sideways with the appropriate ear uppermost, or the head should be tilted to the side.
- Gently pull the pinna backwards and downwards in children under 3 years, and upwards and backwards in older children, to straighten the ear canal.
- Administer the prescribed amount of drops into the ear canal and then gently massage the tragus to help move the drops down the ear.
- The child should keep the ear upwards for five minutes to allow the medication to drain down the ear canal.
- Wash your hands and document in the same way as for other medication.

Transdermal administration

A number of drugs can be administered transdermally, including local anaesthetics to reduce the pain of procedures (EMLA and Ametop). The main advantage of the transdermal route is that it is relatively painless. Corticosteroid creams are used for the treatment of inflammatory conditions of the skin (other than those caused by infection). Fentanyl patches are designed to mimic the delivery achieved with continuous intravenous infusion, for the treatment of children with chronic pain.

Remember that the potential for toxic effects using the transdermal route in children is high due to the variation in blood flow and due to thinner skin and larger body surface area. Care must be taken to prevent accidental absorption through mucous membranes (should the child suck on the medication or rub it into the eye).

Transdermal administration technique

When administering medication via the transdermal route, always follow the manufacturer's guidelines and instructions for use. As with any other medication, you should check contra-indications and allergies before application. In general, you should apply to clean, dry, unbroken, non-irritated, non-irradiated, non-hairy skin. Avoid applying excess medication, and application to damaged skin and mucosal surfaces. Throughout the period of application children should be carefully observed to ensure that they do not ingest the medicine by sucking or chewing. Fentanyl patches should be applied to the torso or upper arm and removed after 72 hours. Replacement patches should be sited in a different area, avoiding the same site for several days. Remember that some drugs, such as Fentanyl, which is an opioid analgesic, have a long duration of action. Children may need to be monitored for up to 24 hours after patch removal. Used patches should be disposed of carefully to prevent accidental ingestion.

The following case study emphasises the importance of taking care with potentially toxic local anaesthetics.

Case study

A 7½-month-old girl died following administration of tetracaine/adrenaline/cocaine (TAC) solution for local wound anaesthesia. The infant died several hours after being discharged from hospital. A 10mL dose of the TAC solution inappropriately came into contact with the nasal mucous membranes, causing excessive drug absorption. The infant's death was probably due to cocaine toxicity as post-mortem blood levels were excessive (Dailey, 1988).

The last route of administration we are looking at is the inhaled route. You will often be asked to administer medicines to children by this route, and to explain to parents how this is done at home.

The inhaled route

The mucosal lining of the respiratory tract provides a large surface area for drug absorption and is useful for the treatment of pulmonary conditions such as asthma, and for the delivery of drugs to other areas via the circulatory system. Mucosal surfaces are rich in blood supply, providing the means for rapid drug absorption into the systemic circulation. Administration can be by inhalation of powder, vapour, and aerosol or nebulised drugs. Drugs administered by this route include bronchodilators, corticosteroids, antibiotics, and antifungal and antiviral agents. Inhaled medications are only effective if they are administered correctly, in order for the drug to reach the lungs. The mouth should be rinsed with water following inhalation of corticosteroids to prevent oral thrush.

Inhaled route administration technique

Inhaler devices for the treatment of chronic asthma

Children under 5 years

National Institute for Health and Clinical Evidence (NICE) guidelines (2000) recommend that, for children under the age of 5 years, both corticosteroid and bronchodilator therapy should be routinely delivered by pressurised metered dose inhalers (pMDIs) and a spacer device with a face mask where necessary. Spacer devices hold the medicine in a chamber after the drug has been released from the pMDI, allowing the medicine to be inhaled more slowly and deeply. Spacers reduce the amount of medicine deposited in the mouth and increase the amount of medicine reaching the lungs. Spacers eliminate the need for the child to time the release of medication with inhalation. Larger-sized spacers appear to be more effective than smaller ones. Nebulised therapy may be considered depending on the child's clinical condition and where the combination of pMDI and spacer and mask is not effective. It is generally considered that large-volume spacer devices are as effective as a nebuliser for treating mild and moderate exacerbations of asthma (BTS/SIGN, 2008).

Dry powder inhalers may be considered in children aged 3–5 years.

Children from birth to 2 years
Avoid breath-actuated and dry powder inhalers.

Children aged 5–15 years
A pMDI and suitable spacer device is recommended as the first choice for the delivery of inhaled corticosteroids. However, where the adherence to this combination is likely to be poor, alternative devices should be considered. For drugs other than inhaled corticosteroids (such as bronchodilators), it is recommended that a wider range of devices be considered due to the need for more frequent and spontaneous use, and for portability. In the case of bronchodilators, the device user should get a relief of symptoms as feedback that they have used the device correctly. Inhaler devices chosen should be based on therapeutic need, the child's preference, ability to learn an effective technique and suitability for the child and carer's lifestyle.

How to use a metered dose inhaler

Each inhaler device will have specific manufacturer's instruction for use and the following are general instructions.

When using a pMDI for the first time (or if it has not been used for two weeks or more) the inhaler will need to be primed. Shake the canister for five seconds, remove the cap and press down on the canister with the index finger four times to release the medication. The child should be standing or sitting up straight to ensure full diaphragmatic expansion. Make sure the child's chin is lifted upwards to open the airways. Remove the cap from the mouthpiece and shake the canister to mix the medication. Ask the child to breathe out fully and place the mouthpiece in the mouth between the teeth without biting it. Ask the child to breathe in slowly and deeply through the mouthpiece and, simultaneously, you should press the canister to release one puff of medication. Ask the child to hold the breath for 10 seconds. If a second dose of medication is required, wait 30–60 seconds and shake the canister before asking the child to take a second puff. Replace the cap.

How to use a metered dose inhaler with spacer and face mask

The child should be standing or sitting up straight to ensure full diaphragmatic expansion, and the chin is lifted upwards to open the airways. Remove the cap from the mouthpiece and shake the canister to mix the medication. Attach the inverted canister to the spacer and mask device. Place the face mask over the child's nose and mouth, ensuring a good seal, and press the canister to release one puff of medication. Ensure that the one-way valve in the spacer device falls open by gently tilting upwards 45 degrees. Leave the mask in place while the child takes at least six breaths. Allow 30–60 seconds before repeating the full sequence in order to give a second puff (the canister must be shaken again to avoid a dose containing mostly propellant).

How to use a metered dose inhaler and spacer with mouthpiece

The child should be standing or sitting up straight to ensure full diaphragmatic expansion and the chin is lifted upwards to open the airways. Remove the cap from the mouthpiece and shake the canister to mix the medication. Attach the inverted canister to the spacer device. Place the mouthpiece in the child's mouth between the teeth, tongue down and sealed with lips. Press the canister to release one puff of medication. Encourage the child to breathe in and out gently for five or six breaths, ensuring that the valve opens and closes by listening for the clicking noise. Allow 30–60 seconds before repeating the full sequence in order to give a second puff (remove the canister and shake again to disperse the medication).

Cleaning the spacer

A build-up of electrostatic charge causes the drug to stick to the inside surface and reduces drug delivery. Wash the device monthly in detergent and allow it to air dry. Washing more frequently and in water alone causes electrostatic charge to develop, reducing the effectiveness of the spacer. Replace the device every 6–12 months.

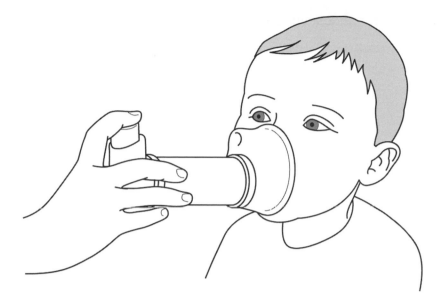

Figure 6.9: Using a metered dose inhaler with an infant

Cleaning the pressurised metered dose inhaler

It is important to clean the aerosol spray port to prevent clogging and clean the mouthpiece of medication particles. Remove the metal canister from the plastic sleeve and wash the sleeve in warm water. Dry thoroughly before reusing. Do not submerge or wash the metal canister as water can damage the valve system.

Dry powder inhalers

Dry powder inhalers (DPIs) are usually suitable for children over about 5 years of age as they require the child's respiratory effort to disperse the medication. Some school-aged children may prefer these devices and may find them easier to use than pMDIs, with less irritation. The disadvantage is that they cannot be used with spacer devices. A Turbohaler is an easy-to-use dry powder format. Some Turbohalers feature a dose counter that shows the exact amount of medication left.

How to use a Turbohaler

Unscrew and remove the cap and hold the inhaler upright. Twist the coloured grip of the Turbohaler as far as it will go. Then twist it all the way back. You should hear a 'click'. The child should breathe out gently. Encourage the child to place the mouthpiece between the teeth, and seal the lips around it. The child should then breathe in forcefully and deeply through the mouth. Remove the inhaler from the mouth before asking the child to breathe out. Replace the cap.

If the device is dropped or breathed into after the dose has been loaded, the dose will be lost and you need to reload. The device must be kept dry as it will not work properly if it gets wet. It can be cleaned by wiping the mouthpiece with a dry tissue.

Ensuring that the inhaler device is not empty

You must be sure, when you are administering medication from any inhaler device, that there are sufficient doses within it. It is not possible to determine if a pMDI inhaler is empty by shaking it, as some propellant remains in the canister even when the medication is gone. Some inhalers have counter devices to track the amount of medication used. For those devices that do not have a counter you will need to keep track of how many doses are available and when a refill will be needed. It is a good idea to write the date the canister will need to be refilled in permanent marker on the inhaler. For relievers that are used infrequently it is more difficult to determine when they are empty. The package should indicate the number of puffs or sprays available in the inhaler, which can be divided by the number of average puffs per month.

The following activity should help you to calculate the replacement of regularly used inhaler devices.

Activity 6.6   *Evidence-based practice and research*

Four-year-old Gemma is prescribed beclomethasone dipropionate 200 micrograms twice daily as regular inhaled preventer therapy for chronic asthma. Gemma takes her medication via a pMDI and spacer device. The aerosol inhaler 100 micrograms/metered inhalation 200 dose unit was commenced on 1st March.

* Around what date will Gemma need a refill for her device?

An outline answer is provided at the end of the chapter.

The following activity should help you to calculate the replacement of infrequently used inhaler devices.

Activity 6.7   *Evidence-based practice and research*

Gemma occasionally uses the short-acting beta 2 agonist salbutamol for relief of her asthma symptoms. She is prescribed 100–200 micrograms (1–2) puffs up to four times daily as needed. On average she would need to take two puffs of this inhaler no more than once per week. She started a new salbutamol metered dose inhaler 200 units on 1st April.

* Around what date will Gemma need a refill for her device?

An outline answer is provided at the end of the chapter.

Nebuliser administration

Nebulisers deliver medicines in the form of a vapour that can be breathed in through a mask or mouthpiece. The nebuliser machine uses compressed gas or vibration to aerosolise liquids. They are sometimes used in the treatment of severe or life-threatening asthma to deliver bronchodilators with oxygen. They can also be used for the administration of inhaled corticosteroid in severe croup and to deliver the antibacterial tobramycin for cystic fibrosis.

Nebuliser administration technique

Preparation

Each child must have his or her own nebuliser, tubing and mouthpiece or mask to avoid cross-infection. Mouthpieces are more effective than masks as the aerosol solution can be lost through the mask vents. The medication may require dilution before administration if the volume is too small to ensure adequate vapour formation. Nebulisers need to be driven by a gas, which is indicated by the prescriber and which can be air or oxygen. Remember that all oxygen should be prescribed. In acute asthma, the driving gas should be oxygen. The driving gas flow rate is very important and influences the nebulisation time and the size of droplets being dispersed. For efficient drug delivery, gas flow rate should be 6–8L/min (BTS, 1997).

The recommended diluent is sterile sodium chloride 0.9%. Check the prescription and nebuliser manufacturer's instructions for minimum volumes. The usual minimum volume should be 4mL for it to work properly, maximum 10mL (BTS, 1997).

Plug the nebuliser compressor into the mains and connect the tubing between the compressor and mouthpiece or mask. Place the medication into the nebuliser chamber and replace the top before attaching to the face mask or mouthpiece (check with the pharmacist before mixing medications in the chamber).

Administration

Ensure that the child is positioned comfortably, preferably upright, to aid diaphragmatic expansion. Place the face mask over the mouth and nose, and secure with the strap. A mouthpiece should be positioned between the teeth and sealed with the lips. The nebuliser chamber must be kept upright to prevent the solution spilling into the tubing. Switch the compressor unit on and encourage the child to breathe as normal; use distractions such as reading a story to them. Children using a mouthpiece should be encouraged to breathe through the mouth, not the nose. During administration any large droplets of the solution on the sides of the chamber should be tapped back down into the solution. Administration should be completed within ten minutes when no more mist is being formed, or one minute after it starts to 'splutter' (BTS, 1997). Switch off the compressor and disconnect the chamber; it is normal for a small amount of solution to be left. Record that the medication has been administered on the drug chart.

Cleaning and care of equipment

It is important that the nebuliser equipment is kept clean and dry to prevent bacterial growth and infection. After each use the nebuliser chamber, mask or mouthpiece should be washed in warm soapy water, rinsed and left to air dry. If the tubing is damp inside, attach it to the compressor and deliver some air through the tubing to dry it out. Wipe over the compressor weekly with a clean damp cloth and dry. Replace the tubing, chamber, mouthpiece and face masks every three months. Replace the compressor filters every three months and ensure that the compressor is serviced annually. To prevent cross-infection separate compressors should be used for those patients colonised with Pseudomonas aeruginosa or Burkholderia cepacia (common in children with cystic fibrosis). After use the air filter should be changed, by returning the compressor to Medical Electronics.

Nasal administration

The nasal route can be used to deliver drugs to have a local effect (beclometasone for allergic rhinitis) or a systemic effect (sumatriptan for migraine, and hormones such as desmopressin acetate for diabetes insipidus). The nasal cavity is well vascularised and drugs are absorbed rapidly through the thin nasal mucosa into the systemic blood system. Nasal medications can be administered in the form of drops, aqueous spray pumps and powdered nasal sprays

Nasal drops administration technique

Check that the prescription is correct and states the number of drops, one or both nostrils, and the route and drug strength. Nasal drops should be marked with the name of the child for individual use to prevent cross-infection. Clean the child's nose of any secretions first by blowing the nose with a tissue or use a gauze swab. Wash your hands. Position the child comfortably with the head tilted backwards over the edge of a bed or with the neck hyperextended by placing a rolled blanket under the shoulders. Shake the bottle and place as many drops as prescribed into the nostril, squeezing the bottle gently to allow the drops to fall. Then sit the child up and tilt the head forward to prevent the drops trickling to the back of the throat. If required, repeat for the other nostril. Wash your hands and sign the drug chart.

Nasal spray administration technique

This technique is similar to that for nasal drops, but the child's head should be positioned upright and tilted slightly forward. Close off the opposite nostril by asking the child or parent to press with their finger. Keeping the bottle upright, insert the tip of the spray into the open nostril. Ask the child to breathe in and squirt one spray into the nostril as they inhale. Remove the spray from the nose and ask the child to breathe out through the mouth.

Anaphylaxis

Anaphylaxis is a systemic hypersensitivity reaction that is severe and life-threatening (Resuscitation Council UK, 2008). Anaphylactic shock can occur as a result of the administration of medicines. It is essential, before you administer any medicines likely to cause a reaction, that you check that resuscitation equipment is available and in working order. Anaphylaxis is more likely to occur following intravenous and intramuscular administration of medicines. Medicines particularly associated with anaphylaxis include vaccines, antibacterials, non-steroidal anti-inflammatory medicines (NSAIDs), blood products, allergen immunotherapy drugs and muscle relaxants used in anaesthesia.

The equipment that should be available before drugs are administered, both in hospital and in the community are:

- oxygen and suction;
- adrenaline 1mL syringes, orange and blue needles;
- antihistamines;
- hydrocortisone.

Recognising anaphylactic shock

The signs and symptoms may vary but usually include life-threatening airway and breathing problems and circulation problems associated with skin and mucous membrane changes. Table 6.1 lists the common and less common signs and symptoms.

The treatment of anaphylaxis

Treatment is based on early recognition that the child is seriously ill and on life-support principles. Symptoms can develop within minutes. In general, the more rapid the onset of symptoms, the more serious the reaction will be (Resuscitation Council UK, 2008).

The following treatment must be given immediately.

- Call for help straightaway.
- Use ABCDE: airway, breathing, circulation, disability, exposure.
- For hypotension, lie the child flat with the legs raised.
- Give oxygen if available.
- Administer an age-appropriate dose of adrenaline 1:1000 intramuscularly (anterolateral aspect of the middle third of the thigh) as local protocol.

Frequency	Sign/symptom
Common	Difficulty breathing Hypotension (leading to cardiovascular collapse) Pale or flushed appearance Urticaria (itchy rash with weals) Angioedema (sudden severe swelling of eyes, lips, nose, tongue, larynx, hands, bowel) Sense of impending doom
Less common	Diarrhoea and/or vomiting Rhinitis or conjunctivitis Abdominal pain

Table 6.1: Signs and symptoms of anaphylactic shock

- Repeat the dose of adrenaline in five minutes if no improvement.
- Start CPR in the absence of signs of life or normal breathing.
- Administer prescribed intramuscular hydrocortisone for severe reaction.
- Transfer to hospital by ambulance from community settings.
- Administer antihistamine as prescribed intramuscularly.
- Inhaled salbutamol can be prescribed for severe bronchospasm.

Reporting medication errors

Nurses and other healthcare professionals have a legal and ethical responsibility to report medication errors. You must make yourself aware of local policies and procedures for doing so. You must also be aware of your professional body's guidance for medicines management (NMC, 2010b). It is believed that many medicine errors made by nurses go unreported for fear of reprisals. However, it is impossible to identify and put right faulty systems if nurses fail to report errors. You must also report near misses as well as actual errors so that any necessary changes can be made in the future to improve patient safety. The consequences of not reporting errors can lead to serious harm to the patient if the mistake is not rectified. It is important that employers maintain a culture in which nurses can report drug errors and near misses without fear of reprisal.

Activity 6.8   *Team working*

Student nurse Caitlin O'Boyle was on placement in a busy children's accident and emergency department. Caitlin had been asked by her mentor to assist a Dr Khan in suturing the leg wound of a 6-year-old child called Oscar. Oscar had never been given his preschool booster, which includes tetanus vaccine. As it was considered that he had a tetanus-prone wound, his parent had consented to him being given the diphtheria, tetanus, pertussis and polio booster (DtaP/IPV) in the department. The staff nurse and the student nurse had already checked and prepared the booster together. When they approached Oscar with the injection, Dr Khan was with him and was preparing to suture the wound. The staff nurse placed the vaccine at the end of the bed in the receiver and asked the student nurse to look after it until Dr Khan had finished. Before Caitlin could stop him, Dr Khan picked up the booster injection and injected it into Oscar's wound. Dr Khan had assumed that the staff nurse had prepared some local anaesthetic for him to inject into the wound prior to suturing. Caitlin asked Dr Khan to come away from the patient to discuss what had happened with him and the staff nurse. When Dr Khan and the staff nurse were informed of the mistake, they told Caitlin not to tell anyone else and they would sort it out. Caitlin was worried about this as she didn't want to get anyone into trouble. However, she knew it was wrong to cover up the mistake and informed the senior nurse. The consultant was informed and the registrar and staff nurse were reprimanded for asking a student nurse to keep quiet about it. No serious harm occurred to Oscar. The members of staff involved were asked to write an incident report and statement about the error.

continued opposite . . .

continued . . . .

Now answer the following questions.

- Could the error be attributed to a possible failure in the system?
- What mistakes did the staff nurse make?
- What mistakes did the registrar make?
- Could the error have been prevented?

Outline answers are provided at the end of the chapter.

Adverse drug reactions

An adverse drug reaction is an unwanted or harmful reaction following the administration of a medicine. This may be a new and previously unrecognised reaction, or it may be a known side effect of the medicine. You have a responsibility to report the adverse reaction using the Yellow Card Scheme. Yellow Cards are available at the back of the BNFC, or you can complete the form online at **www.yellowcard.gov.uk**.

Chapter summary

This chapter has covered the procedures for the safe administration of medicines to children. You should now be able to interpret a prescription chart correctly and should be aware of the documentation necessary for the administration of medicines. The checks necessary before, during and after administration have been discussed. The chapter has discussed some of the different routes and methods of administration of medicines. It has discussed the use of enteral feeding tubes; however, you need to research further into the use of other equipment such as syringe pumps and drivers. You must always follow local policy and procedure when using equipment. You should now be able to recognise anaphylaxis and how to manage the condition. Recognising and reporting adverse drug reactions has been briefly mentioned. The Medicine and Healthcare Products Regulatory Agency (MHRA) website is provided at the end of the chapter for further information.

Activities: brief outline answers

Activity 6.1 Contraindications for salicylic acid paint (page 135)

Before administering the salicylic acid paint to Charlotte's toes, you should check the BNFC where you will see that this medicine is contraindicated for children under 5 years. Do not be more relaxed when administering topical applications to children than you would be with other routes. Salicylate toxicity can occur if the medication is applied to large areas of skin. This medicine is not licensed for children under 5 years and you would be accountable for your actions if you administered it.

Activity 6.2 Verbal order of a prescriber (page 136)

Remember that there must be a legal prescription before anyone can administer medication. You may, under certain circumstances, be asked to administer a medicine on a verbal order, perhaps taken over the telephone. In order to ensure patient safety, verbal orders may only be taken in an emergency. Remember that you are accountable for your actions and you must be able to justify that the situation was an emergency. A verbal order must contain the same information as a written order to be valid. You must document the verbal instructions, including the date and time, and if possible have the instructions witnessed by a colleague. The verbal instructions should include drug name, dose, route and frequency. The prescriber must write up and sign for the verbal order within 24 hours.

Activity 6.3 Patient specific direction (page 138)

The drug was prescribed to be given on 20 October 2010. As it was a pre-anaesthetic medication, the prescriber could not be specific about the time as they were not aware of the time the child would be going to theatre. It was up to the clinical judgement of the nurse administering the medication as to what time to administer the dose, which needs to be 1–2 hours before the anaesthetic.

The prescriber has written the brand name 'Vallergan' – the correct prescription would have been written as 'alimemazine tartrate'.

Activity 6.4 Patient specific direction (page 139)

- The route of administration for the amoxicillin is oral (PO).
- The prescription is for five days, which means that the last dose should be administered at 0600 on 8th April.
- The 'V' stands for patient vomiting as a reason why the dose was not administered at 1400 on 5th April .

Activity 6.5 Intramuscular administration (page 151)

Morphine sulphate is not a large-volume injection. You should offer James a choice of sites between the upper outer aspect of his non-injured arm and the lateral aspect of the thigh. The middle of the front of the thigh is much more painful, so is not a first choice. Buttocks can have reduced absorption and it is likely that James would be reluctant to expose this area.

Activity 6.6 Refill of beclomethasone dipropionate inhaler (page 158)

If Gemma is prescribed 200 micrograms beclomethasone dipropionate twice daily, she will be given two puffs of the inhaler twice per day to administer the dose. This would mean she is given four doses per day. The inhaler contains 200 doses. Therefore, to calculate the number of days the inhaler would last, divide 200 units by 4.

$$200 \div 4 = 50$$

The inhaler device would last for 50 days. It was commenced on 1st March, so would need to be replaced by 19th April.

Activity 6.7 Refill of salbutamol inhaler (page 158)

Gemma is on average using only eight puffs (8 units) per month, so the inhaler would last for about 25 months. However, you must check the manufacturer's expiry dates for each inhaler as, once opened, some expire after 3–6 months.

Activity 6.8 Covering up a medication error (pages 162–3)

When health professionals realise they have made a mistake, they may panic and try to cover up the incident. It is important that you realise that you have not committed a crime but have made a mistake. It is important that mistakes are not blown up out of proportion.

The policy for administration of medicines within the accident and emergency department should be reviewed, but it is likely that the mistake occurred because the staff nurse and registrar were not adhering to policy. Following guidelines minimises risk.

The staff nurse should never have prepared a medicine and then left it unattended and unlabelled in the department. She asked the student nurse to 'look after it' but this was unacceptable. As the registered nurse she is accountable for the safe-keeping and administration of the medicine. The staff nurse should never have tried to cover up her mistake or the mistake of another health professional.

The registrar should never have administered a medicine he had not prepared and checked himself. Ultimately, he was responsible for his actions and should have immediately reported the error to his senior doctor and informed Oscar's parents.

The mistake could have been prevented by the healthcare professionals being less complacent and following procedure. The staff nurse should have interrupted the doctor and administered the injection right away. If it was not possible to give the injection immediately, she should have labelled the injection and locked it away in a medicine cupboard until she could administer it.

Further reading

Nursing and Midwifery Council (NMC) (2007) *Standards for Medicines Management.* London: Nursing and Midwifery Council. Available online at www.nmc-uk.org/aDisplayDocument.aspx?Document ID=3251.

These are the Nursing and Midwifery Council's guidelines for safe practice and the administration of medicines by registered nurses, midwives and specialist community public health nurses.

Useful websites

www.bapen.org.uk/res_drugs.html

The British Association for Parenteral and Enteral Nutrition (BAPEN) aims to ensure that patients suffering with nutritional problems are appropriately recognised and managed. BAPEN has developed information resources on the administration of drugs via enteral feeding tubes.

www.mhra.gov.uk/index.htm

The Medicine and Healthcare products Regulatory Agency (MHRA) provides safety information on medical devices in order to safeguard the health of the public. This includes drug safety updates.

Chapter 7
Working in partnership with parents, carers and children in medicines management

NMC Standards for Pre-registration Nursing Education

This chapter will address the following competencies:

Domain 2: Communication and interpersonal skills

1. All nurses must build partnerships and therapeutic relationships through safe, effective and non-discriminatory communication. They must take account of individual differences, capabilities and needs.

1.1 **Children's nurses** must work with the child, young person and others to ensure that they are actively involved in decision-making, in order to maintain their independence and take account of their ongoing intellectual, physical and emotional needs.

2 All nurses must use a range of communication skills and technologies to support person-centred care and enhance quality and safety. They must ensure people receive all the information they need in a language and manner that allows them to make informed choices and share decision making. They must recognise when language interpretation or other communication support is needed and know how to obtain it.

2.1 **Children's nurses** must understand all aspects of development from infancy to young adulthood, and identify each child or young person's developmental stage, in order to communicate effectively with them. They must use play, distraction and communication tools appropriate to the child's or young person's stage of development, including for those with sensory or cognitive impairment.

3. All nurses must use the full range of communication methods, including verbal, non-verbal and written, to acquire, interpret and record their knowledge and understanding of people's needs. They must be aware of their own values and beliefs and the impact this may have on their communication with others. They must take account of the many different ways in which people communicate and how these may be influenced by ill health, disability and other factors, and be able to recognise and respond effectively when a person finds it hard to communicate.

3.1 **Children's nurses** must ensure that, where possible, children and young people understand their healthcare needs and can make or contribute to informed choices about all aspects of their care.

4. All nurses must recognise when people are anxious or in distress and respond effectively, using therapeutic principles, to promote their wellbeing, manage personal safety and

continued opposite . . .

continued . . .

resolve conflict. They must use effective communication strategies and negotiation techniques to achieve best outcomes, respecting the dignity and human rights of all concerned. They must know when to consult a third party and how to make referrals for advocacy, mediation or arbitration.

5. All nurses must use therapeutic principles to engage, maintain and, where appropriate, disengage from professional caring relationships, and must always respect professional boundaries.

6. All nurses must take every opportunity to encourage health-promoting behaviour through education, role modelling and effective communication.

7. All nurses must maintain accurate, clear and complete records, including the use of electronic formats, using appropriate and plain language.

8. All nurses must respect individual rights to confidentiality and keep information secure and confidential in accordance with the law and relevant ethical and regulatory frameworks, taking account of local protocols. They must also actively share personal information with others when the interests of safety and protection override the need for confidentiality.

NMC Essential Skills Clusters

This chapter will address the following ESCs:

Cluster: Medicines management

39. People can trust a newly registered graduate nurse to keep and maintain accurate records using information technology, where appropriate, within a multi-disciplinary framework as a leader and as part of a team and in a variety of care settings including at home.

By the second progression point:

1. Demonstrates awareness of roles and responsibilities within the multi disciplinary team for medicines management, including how and in what ways information is shared within a variety of settings.

By entry to the register:

2. Effectively keep records of medication administered and omitted, in a variety of care settings, including controlled drugs, and ensures others do the same.

40. People can trust a newly registered graduate nurse to work in partnership with people receiving medical treatments and their carers.

By the second progression point:

1. Under supervision involves people and carers in administration and self-administration of medicines.

continued overleaf . . .

continued . . . .

By entry to the register:

2. Works with people and carers to provide clear and accurate information.

3. Gives clear instruction and explanation and checks that the person understands the use of medicines and treatment options.

4. Assesses the person's ability to safely self-administer their medicines.

5. Assists people to make safe and informed choices about their medicines.

Chapter aims

By the end of this chapter, you should be able to:

* understand how to work effectively in partnership with children and young people and parents or carers;

* assist children and young people and parents or carers to make safe and informed choices about their medicines;

* safely and effectively keep records of medicines administered using paper and electronic records;

* understand capacity and demonstrate knowledge of the law regarding consent to treatment;

* assess a child's or young person's ability, and that of their parent or carer, to self-administer medicines.

Case study

A young person came to see me about the rash on her torso that had developed after frequent sunbed use. The GP had seen her previously and had diagnosed a yeast infection, prescribing an antifungal shampoo to be applied every day for five days. The young person was upset as the rash had not cleared, despite the fact that she had followed the treatment by using the antifungal medication to shampoo her hair every day. She had not realised that she should have applied the shampoo to the affected area on her body. Although amusing, we cannot really blame the patient as she had not been given clear enough instructions.

I am only too aware of how easily lack of instructions can lead to misunderstandings. On my very first ward placement as a student nurse I was given a tube of cream and told to 'apply it to Freddie's rash'. Freddie was a 10-month-old infant admitted with measles and was covered head to toe in a measles rash. I dutifully entered the cubicle and smothered him all over in the cream. When the consultant entered the cubicle to examine him, Freddie slid out of his hands. The consultant was quite perplexed as to why someone had applied nappy rash cream all over Freddie's body.

Thankfully, in both of the above stories there was no real harm done. You may have heard other stories, such as the child who was told he had diabetes who thought he was going to 'die of the beasties', as he did not have the ability yet to understand the medical term.

Introduction

Communication is a fundamental skill of the children's nurse and you must learn to communicate effectively with children of all ages as well as their families in order to practise safely. As a children's nurse you must aim to work with children and young people to ensure that they are actively involved in decisions about their care (NMC, 2010a). Partnership working, building therapeutic relationships and enabling children and young people and their families to remain in control of their healthcare form the ethos of child nursing. This concept will be explored in the context of medicines management. Partnership working, communication and child development are extensive subjects and the content of this chapter is far from inclusive. It is recommended that you use this chapter as a foundation and seek out further resources on the subjects. There is more discussion of these issues in Chapter 3.

Record keeping is fundamental to safe and effective practice. You must learn how to keep effective records of medication administered and omitted in a variety of settings. Many healthcare settings now use electronic as well as paper-based records. The principles of good record keeping are included here.

The subject of consent to medical treatment concerning children and young people is complex. It is hoped that this chapter will provide you with enough information to understand the law and begin to make decisions in practice.

Partnership working

As a children's nurse you have a duty to acknowledge and understand the unique role of the family, and the rights and responsibilities of parents and carers. It is important to encourage active participation and involve families when planning and delivering care. Partnership working involves the concept of equality in relation to decision making. As a registered nurse you should be competent to provide care and advice in the area of medicines administration. However, the parents and family can contribute their unique knowledge and experience of the child to enhance that care. Parents need to feel valued and respected in order for effective partnerships to work. The partnership approach to medicine prescribing and taking is known as **concordance**, and differs from 'compliance', which is following instructions. Concordance recognises that people make their own decisions about taking medicines and have a right to decline them after being informed of the benefits and risks. Nurses must participate in respectful negotiation with children/young people and parents/carers in order to bring into being successful partnership relationships. Mutual trust and respect is crucial to achieving equality in relationships and a balance of power. Children/young people and parents/carers are more likely to be committed to taking their medicines if they have been fully involved in the decision making about their treatment.

The following activity is to help you to think about the importance of partnership working.

Activity 7.1 *Communication*

Ruby is 4 years old and has been admitted to an acute paediatric ward for the second time in two months with an acute exacerbation of asthma. Ruby's mum, Sally, admitted that she sometimes forgot to give Ruby her steroid inhaler when she was at home. Sally had been administering Ruby's salbutamol inhaler as required when Ruby was wheezy. You establish a rapport with Sally and ask her how she feels about Ruby's medicines. Sally discloses that she can see the point of the salbutamol as it actually makes a difference when Ruby is unwell. However, she didn't really seem to think the steroid made any difference to Ruby when she was well and not wheezy. Also, she didn't like giving medicine unnecessarily to Ruby and had heard bad things about the side effects of steroids.

- What should you do in this situation?

An outline answer is provided at the end of the chapter.

Involving children and young people in decision making

Children and young people should be involved in decisions about their care. The United Nations Convention on the Rights of the Child (UN General Assembly, 1989) clearly advocated the rights of every child to self-determination and the right to make informed decisions. The National Service Framework for Children (DH, 2003) emphasises this principle by stating that children should be active partners in their care. Children's nurses should give the child or young person explanations of treatments such as medicines and their options. Their views should be taken into account and they should be encouraged to participate in decisions that affect them appropriate to their age and understanding. The level of participation will vary depending on the decision being made, and the age and capability of the child. You should act as an advocate for the child or young person and ensure that your actions support their equality, diversity and rights. Children with complex needs or with communication or learning difficulties should also be given the opportunity to be involved in the decision-making process. Strategies should be devised in order to establish their views (DH, 1991). Do not assume that disabled children and young people are incapable of being involved in decision making.

Self-administration of medicines

Patient self-administration means that patients administer their own medicine while in hospital under the supervision of nursing staff. Children's wards have been slower than adult areas to implement this practice. Self-administration of medicines should be encouraged and supported (NMC, 2004). Self-administration has many advantages, including allowing the child/young person and parents/carers to become familiar with their medicines in a safe environment and identifying any problems before discharge. It may also increase concordance and increase their understanding and knowledge of their medication. It allows the child/young person and parents/carers to be involved in their care and make decisions about their medicines. It is also possible for them to establish routines closer to that at home, which is important for medicines such as insulin. Anecdotal evidence suggests that it may also reduce medication errors and may save nursing time as once established the workload is reduced.

However, agreed procedures must be in place beforehand to ensure that safe administration and storage policies are adhered to. Before delegating the responsibility, the registered nurse should ensure that the child/young person or parent/carer is competent to carry out the task. Self-administration is not suitable for all children/young people and parents/carers and some may not want to undertake it. Not all medications are always suitable, for example intravenous drugs or controlled drugs will not be self-administered. Education, training and assessment must take place before self-administration is set up and this can be time-consuming.

There are different levels of supervision when practising self-administration on the ward. Full self-administration is where the child/young person and parents/carers administer the medicine themselves without any supervision and have responsibility for the key to their drug locker. Close supervision applies where the child/young person and parents/carers have to request their medication from the nursing staff at appropriate times and check it with the nurses.

The following activity will help you to think about supporting children/young people and parents/carers to safely self-administer medication.

Activity 7.2 — *Decision making*

What levels of self-administration would you assess as suitable for the following children/young people on an acute paediatric ward?

- Sophie is 14 years old and has insulin-dependent diabetes mellitus. She has been administering her own insulin at home for seven years. She is willing to continue self-administering. Sophie has been admitted to the ward for some non-invasive investigations.
- Jessica is 14 years old and has been admitted to the ward for a tonsillectomy under general anaesthesia. She has a history of being admitted following a paracetamol overdose six months ago, but she recovered well and has normal liver function. She is prescribed co-codamol for pain following the operation.

Outline answers are provided at the end of the chapter.

Communicating with children/young people and their families

Good communication is essential to effective partnership working with children/young people, families and carers. Communicating effectively builds trust, and ensures that active participation in care takes place. Communication is an active process that involves listening, questioning, understanding and responding. The nurse's role in communicating is not just to inform children and families about their treatment, but to create a therapeutic relationship. You should always communicate with children and young people in a way that matches their developmental stage, needs and individual circumstances.

Case study

Carole, a third-year children's nursing student, recalled an incident in her first year when a doctor had asked her to assist him to insert a cannula into a 3-year-old girl. The doctor was not experienced in paediatrics, English was his second language, which made him difficult to understand, and he was from a different culture. Carole observed that the doctor did not speak to the child or the mother to give an explanation or gain consent for the procedure. His eye contact was poor and his body language aggressive. When the child became distressed, he shouted at the child to be quiet and asked Carole to hold the child still. Both parent and child were visually distressed. Carole appropriately stopped the procedure and went to her mentor for advice and assistance in dealing with the situation.

- *What could the doctor have done better in this situation?*

The doctor was obviously inexperienced in dealing with young children and their carers and needed some guidance and support. He should have first established a rapport with the child and the mother by greeting them appropriately and introducing himself. Before attempting to go ahead with the cannulation, he should have fully explained the reason for the procedure with the mother and obtained her consent. The child should not be ignored, regardless of age. He should have explained the procedure to the child using language she could understand and showing empathy and care. It is important to make sure at all times that you are fully understood by children/young people and their parents/carers. The child and mother should have been made to feel at ease, which they were not. The doctor's clarity of speech, eye contact and general approach to the situation were poor.

Communicating with children and young people of different ages

As a children's nurse you must develop the knowledge and skills needed in order to communicate effectively with children and young people of different ages. It is not possible to be specific about developmental milestones as these differ from child to child. When communicating with children you need to take into consideration their social, emotional and language developmental stages as well as their intellectual ability. You will gain the skills to do this from experience and by observing more experienced colleagues.

Infants

The primary method of communicating with infants is non-verbally. Infants respond best to confident but gentle handling and a calm voice. Older infants from about seven months onwards will have anxiety towards strangers. Parents are best kept in the child's view.

Preschool age children (2–5 years)

At this age children see the world only from their own perspective and only their own experience is relevant. It is no use trying to get them to cooperate by demonstrating another child's behaviour. For example, 'Look at Fiona, she is taking her medicine' won't work. You need to be direct, concrete and literal, for example, 'Open your mouth, Hamid, and I will put this tablet on your tongue so you can swallow it.' Use short, simple questions and take time to give explanations for unfamiliar equipment.

School-age children (6–12 years)

School-age children are able to see the world in a more complex way. They move from being concrete thinkers to abstract thinking. They want to know how things work and why things are done and should be given explanations, for example, 'Sarah, this tubing puts the medicine into your blood, so your heart will pump it all around your body.'

Adolescents

Adolescents want to be adults but have not yet developed the emotional maturity to achieve this. Sometimes they are capable of mature decisions, but under stress are more likely to respond in a childlike way. You should not treat them as children, but at the same time you cannot assume that their learning ability and communication style can be consistently at an adult level. Adolescents need to feel valued and respected. You must always be honest and open with them otherwise you will lose their trust. The adolescent will require explanations and rationales for things in order to cooperate with you.

The following activity is to help you to think about how you communicate with children of different ages.

Activity 7.3 — *Reflection*

Think about some interactions you have had in practice with children of different ages and ask yourself the following questions.

- Do I frequently have one-to-one conversations with children/young people that allow them time to respond and speak freely about their feelings?
- Do I allow children to make decisions and involve them in the planning of their care?
- Do I always give children age-appropriate explanations for their care?
- Do I sometimes provide false assurances or reassurances about their treatment?

There are no answers to this activity, but you may want to discuss these questions further with your mentor or use them for an entry in your reflective diary.

Non-verbal communication

We communicate not only with words, but also with body language and the way in which we speak. Your appearance sends messages to others and the wearing of a nursing uniform can create positive or negative stereotypes. You need to show empathy and sincerity by such gestures as open body posture and leaning towards the other person. Gestures send messages. Folded arms and legs can be interpreted as defensiveness or disinterest. You must develop self-awareness and be aware how your behaviour and attitude can affect children and their parents.

The face reflects a wide range of emotions. Your own facial expression should reflect a nurse who is interested, sincere and attentive to the child/young person. You should maintain eye contact, but you should not stare and should occasionally glance away. You must also take into account cultural differences and be aware that some cultures avoid direct eye contact. The tones of voice, intensity, pitch and pauses have as much meaning as the words spoken. Patients may use the tone of their voice to show sarcasm or hostility. A touch on the hand or arm can show empathy, but only use this if you know that it will be interpreted correctly.

Activity 7.4   *Reflection*

Your own appearance sends a message to children/young people and parents/carers. Examine your own appearance at work. Do you convey a competent and professional image to others? Look around at your colleagues and other professionals and consider what image they convey. Does your uniform create a positive image that is comforting and easy to identify? Or does your uniform convey authority, formality and create a distance between yourself and the children/young people and parents/carers?

There are no answers to this activity, but you may want to discuss these questions further with your mentor or use them for an entry in your reflective diary.

Culture and communication

The way people communicate with each other differs between cultures and you must have some awareness of this in order to avoid misunderstandings or offending others. In some cultures 'yes' means 'I am attentive' more than 'I agree'. Non-verbal communication can vary significantly, for example finger pointing can be offensive in some cultures. Patting a child on the head as a friendly gesture would be inappropriate for many Asians, who believe that the head is a sacred part of the body. Touch between individuals of opposite genders would be considered inappropriate by some people of Muslim cultures, who may require a nurse of the same gender. What is considered appropriate eye contact within Western culture would be thought to be rude in some Middle Eastern and Asian cultures. The book in this series, *Communication and Interpersonal Skills for Nurses* (Bach and Grant, 2009), has much helpful advice in this area.

English as an additional language

You must always promote conditions that encourage respect for different cultures. If English is an additional language of the child and family, you need to be aware of this and communicate appropriately. Children and carers who are not fluent in English should be offered the services of an interpreter. In order for you to deliver safe and effective healthcare, you must be able to understand the child and carer and be understood by them. If communication is poor, it can be confusing and distressing for families, and dangerous misunderstandings can occur. The use of an approved medical interpreter can help you to communicate clearly and they are bound to communicate the information accurately and in full. Interpreters should have some training or experience of medical terminology, as well as being culturally sensitive and aware of Western health concepts. You should not rely on a family member or family friend to interpret medical information. Family and friends should only be used in an emergency or for non-essential healthcare. Information may be misinterpreted by family or friends as they do not understand it or know how to phrase it in their own language. They may also be embarrassed by the information or trying to protect their relative.

You should ensure that the child and family have access to resources in their own language. The NHS 'Equip' website (see 'Useful websites' at the end of the chapter) provides useful links to resources that offer information in different languages.

Communicating with children and parents with disabilities

Many children and their parents or carers have disabilities that make it difficult for them to communicate. It is essential for you to identify disabilities and adapt your communication style effectively to suit their individual needs. This sometimes means using alternative forms of communication to spoken language, such as information and communication technologies, pictures, play, British Sign Language or Makaton. There are some useful websites for alternative forms of communication at the end of the chapter.

Play as a form of communication

Play has an important role when communicating with children and young people and serves many functions. Most acute paediatric settings now employ a play specialist who is specifically trained to help children understand the hospital experience and support them through the experience. Where there are difficulties with the child refusing or fearing medication, the play specialist can be involved to allow the child to express their fears and fantasies. The play specialist will use various resources, such as teddies, story books, dolls, role play and medical equipment, to help the child understand and take control of the situation (NCB, 2008). There are some useful websites at the end of the chapter.

Individuals with a learning disability

When speaking to children with learning disabilities, you should use simple but not childish words. Ensure that the information you give is clear and precise. You may need to repeat the information and rephrase it in several ways. Use concrete examples. To confirm that the person has understood, ask them to repeat the message back to you.

Individuals with visual impairment

Speak to them in your usual way but avoid using terms such as 'I'll show you how', or 'have you seen . . .?' that refer to sight. Be aware that your hand gestures and facial expressions will not be noticed, so you must always respond verbally to questions. Avoid long pauses in speech and talking louder than normal. Always tell the person where you are and let them know if you are leaving.

Individuals with hearing impairment

Make sure that you have the person's attention before you speak and use your normal speed and tone of voice. Articulate your speech clearly but do not exaggerate it. It is helpful to use gestures such as facial expressions, actions and pictures to aid understanding. Stop frequently to check they have understood and if necessary rephrase and repeat the information. If you find it difficult to understand their speech, show that you are interested and do not hesitate to ask them to repeat themselves. Avoid speaking for them and give them the opportunity to express themselves.

Listening and building empathy

Building relationships takes time and effort. Establish a rapport with the child and family by making them the focus of your attention. Introduce yourself and use their names. Be reliable and do what you say you will do in order to establish trust. Be honest and supportive, but do not make unrealistic promises. If you cannot do something they have asked you to, explain why this is, rather than simply refusing. Hold conversations at the appropriate time and place. Ask how they feel; listen and do not interrupt. Use non-verbal signs such as a head nod to show you are paying attention to what they are saying. Remain calm, open and non-judgemental. Acknowledge what has been said and check that you have understood correctly by summarising and paraphrasing the discussion, for example, 'So you are saying that you think Sarah won't be able to use her insulin pump in hospital, but we need to get her an insulin pen while she is here.'

Self-disclosure can be used with care to show you are human and not just 'a nurse'. For example, if the child has difficulty swallowing tablets, you might disclose that you find it hard to swallow tablets also. Do not get carried away and tell your life story; a few short sentences here and there in order to relate to patients is sufficient. Make the child or family feel valued and care for each one as an individual. To work in partnership you must give the child and parent some control. Provide them with options when you can; for example, ask if they prefer a tablet or liquid medicine. Always explain why you are doing things in lay terms ('this will help you do a poo' rather than 'pass a bowel motion'). Ensure that the child and family know that you are there to support them and that they can ask if they are unsure.

Communicating with team workers

Errors in medicine are frequently due to poor teamwork and poor communication rather than individual mistakes. In order to ensure that medicines are managed effectively it is important that all members of the healthcare team work together. There must be some form of feedback between the nurse, pharmacist, prescriber and other healthcare professionals involved. Any new clinical features that the child/young person develops after the commencement of the medication need to be reported and evaluated, and the medicine continued or changed appropriately. For some children/young people a more collaborative and multidisciplinary approach to treatment will be needed, for example the child with cystic fibrosis who may be receiving many different medicines and therapies. Effective care and evaluation of treatment necessitates ongoing communication between all members of the healthcare team, including pharmacists, physiotherapists, dieticians, paediatricians and nurses. There is more about the roles of other healthcare team members in Chapter 3.

Barriers to effective communication

Be aware that factors such as anxiety, tiredness, illness and stress can hinder effective communication; you need to try to reduce this. Lack of time due to staff shortages or other pressures can hinder communication. Distractions and interruptions, such as the telephone ringing, will create difficulties. Effective communication requires committed attention. Miscommunications can also occur when using medical terminology, idioms or jargon and should be avoided. Differing social norms, generation gaps and accents can also be a barrier to effective communication (Park and Song, 2004).

Record keeping

Good record keeping is an integral part of nursing practice and essential to safe and effective practice (NMC, 2009). The use of electronic record keeping is growing, however paper records are still commonly used in many areas of practice. The principles of good record keeping are the same regardless of the form in which the records are held. A health record is any information about the health of an individual, made by or on behalf of a health professional, in relation to the care of that individual (Data Protection Act 1998). Health records can include electronic notes, handwritten clinical notes, patient medicine administration charts, printouts from monitors, emails, letters between health professionals, incident reports and statements and videos. Good record keeping serves many useful functions, including supporting patient care and communication and improving continuity of care. When administering medications, record keeping serves as the documentary evidence of the medication given. Records can be used to show how decisions were made in relation to medicines administration and to help identify risks such as allergies. Good record keeping can protect you by helping you to deal with complaints or litigation. There is more about record keeping in Chapter 5, and much useful information in *Law and Professional Issues in Nursing* (Griffith and Tengnah, 2010) in this series.

The principles of good record keeping

The reason we keep records is to facilitate communication with colleagues and other health professionals, carry out ongoing assessments and document nursing interventions that have been carried out. Good record keeping increases the likelihood that the child/young person will receive consistent care and decreases the potential for errors.

The following guiding principles are included in the NMC's (2009) *Record Keeping Guidance for Nurses and Midwives*. You should follow this guidance as well as the local policy of your employer.

Handwriting should be legible and all record entries signed with the name, job title, time and date included. Records should be accurate, clear and factual, avoiding unnecessary jargon and abbreviations. You should use your professional judgement when deciding what is relevant and needs to be documented. Details of assessments, reviews, ongoing care and future care plans should be recorded. Information that you have given to parents/carers, children and young people about their care and treatment should be documented. Risks or problems that have been identified should be recorded and the action taken. You must exchange all necessary information about the children in your care with your colleagues. Records must never be destroyed without authorisation, and any alterations made and the original record must remain clear. You must include your name and job title next to alterations and sign and date the original documentation. It is good practice to involve the child/young person and parent/carer in the record-keeping process. Your records should be written in a way that will be easily understood by them. For administration purposes, records should be of sufficient quality to be readable when scanned or photocopied. Never fabricate records or use offensive terms to describe children in your care.

Confidentiality

You must ensure that you are aware of the legal requirements for confidentiality and ensure that you practise in line with local and national policies. You should protect records by ensuring that they are not left unsupervised where they might be seen by others not authorised to do so. Be particularly attentive to computer screens displaying patient records that might be viewed by others.

Access to records

You should inform the children/young people and parents/carers in your care that their health records may be shared with other agencies or professionals involved in their care. You should never access records to find out personal information about an individual unless it is relevant to their care. Children/young people with capacity (see 'Capacity to consent' below) have a right to ask to view their health records, for which local policies should be followed. Children/young people can request that information about them be withheld from health professionals or their parents and this must be respected (unless the withholding of the information would cause serious harm to them or others). Children/young people should not be given information that would cause them harm or any information about another person without the other person's consent. Parents have a right to access their child's notes if the child consents or lacks capacity and it does not go against the child's best interests. If the records contain information given by the child in confidence, it should not be disclosed without their consent. Missing records should be reported to someone in authority and a record kept that you have done so.

> ### Scenario
>
> *Jodie is 15 years old and a patient on your ward; she has had a termination of pregnancy. Her parents are divorced and Jodie lives with her mum, Karen. One evening Jodie's dad, who is a solicitor, visits the ward and asks you for Jodie's nursing and medical notes for him to see, as he would like to know why she has been admitted.*
>
> *What should you do? You are not sure if Jodie's father has parental responsibility as they are divorced. Jodie's father is very authoritative and Jodie is quite subdued in his presence. You have been asked by Jodie not to tell her father the reason she has been admitted.*
>
> *Does Jodie's father have the right to see her nursing and medical notes?*

In the scenario, you should not give Jodie's father access to her nursing or medical records. There is nothing in the law that prevents you from informally showing Jodie her records, but you cannot show them to her father. Parents do not lose parental responsibility through divorce, so Jodie's father still has this and may independently exercise rights of access. Parents may have access to their child's records if it is not against a competent child's wishes. Children over the age of 12 years are generally considered to have sufficient understanding to give or withhold their consent for the release of information from their health records (BMA, 2009). This means that Jodie's consent must be sought before her father can be given access to her nursing or medical records. If Jodie were to consent, her father must make a formal application for access to the records. He must then wait until the health records manager or consultant responsible for Jodie's care decides if the request can be approved. The health records manager or consultant can also refuse Jodie's father access if they believe that releasing the records would be harmful to Jodie's physical or mental health or that of someone else.

Electronic medical records

Electronic records can be used to support patient documentation in many ways. The same principles of paper-based systems of documentation, access, storage and retrieval of records apply. Documentation in electronic health records must also be comprehensive, accurate and timely, and must clearly identify the nurse who provided the information. You should ensure that you are able to use the information systems in use in your practice area. Entries made in an electronic health record are a permanent part of the patient's record and cannot be deleted. You should refer to local policies for correcting documentation errors or making a late entry. You have a duty to protect the confidentiality of your patients' information by maintaining security of the system. Never disclose your password or allow others to access information systems with your identification or authentication details, as this is your electronic signature. Passwords should be changed at frequent intervals and secure passwords that are not easily deciphered should be used. Always ensure that you log out of information systems or close them down when you have finished. Protect patient information displayed on screens by locating them in private areas and using screen savers. Locate printers in secure areas away from public access. You should only access the information that is required to provide nursing care for that patient. Accessing information for any other purpose is a breach of confidentiality.

Consent

It is as important to gain valid consent from children and young people before administering medicines as it is with adults. In some situations the child/young person will be able to give consent themselves; sometimes another person will need to make the decision on their behalf. The following section will go over the main points of gaining consent from children and young people.

The nurse's responsibility

As a children's nurse you have a responsibility to act in the best interests of the child/young person at all times. As previously discussed, you should involve the child/young person in the decisions about their treatments as much as possible, according to their age and level of understanding. If the child/young person is not capable of consenting for themselves, you will need to gain consent from a person with parental responsibility.

Capacity to consent

The legal situation concerning the age at which a person is considered capable of consenting for themselves is complex. It is important that, as a children's nurse, you are clear about the law and consent. The age at which a person is assumed to be an adult and competent to consent or refuse treatment in England, Wales and Northern Ireland is 18 years. When a young person reaches the age of 16 years they are assumed to have the same capacity as an adult to consent to treatment. They do not need parental consent for medical treatments unless there is a reason to believe they lack capacity. As a nurse you have a duty of confidentiality to these young people and you must not disclose information about them to parents without their consent. Children/young people under 18 years cannot give their own consent for blood donations or experimental research unless they have sufficient understanding of what is involved. In Scotland the law differs and the legal age of capacity (the age at which a person is assumed to be an adult) is 16 years.

Activity 7.6   *Decision making*

Georgia is 16 years old and attends a Brook Centre in London as she feels she needs emergency contraception.

- Does Georgia need parental consent for this treatment?

An outline answer is provided at the end of the chapter.

People younger than 16 years

If a child/young person under the age of 16 years can understand the medical treatments being proposed, they are able to consent to that treatment. It is the responsibility of the health professional to decide if the child is capable of understanding the treatment, including the benefits, options and risks. If the child/young person has such understanding, they are considered to be '**Gillick competent**'. In these circumstances the child/young person's parents cannot overrule the child's decision. If the child/young person is not Gillick competent, they cannot give consent or withhold consent for themselves. A person with parental responsibility for the child will need to make the decision on their behalf.

Activity 7.7   *Decision making*

April is 14 years old and attends a Brook Centre in London as she feels she needs emergency contraception and would like to 'go on the pill'.

- Does April need parental consent for this treatment?

An outline answer is provided at the end of the chapter.

Emergency situations

If it is an emergency situation and a person with parental responsibility is not available to give consent, you must act in the child's best interests. Any treatment given should be limited to what is essential to deal with the emergency.

Child/young person refusing consent to treatment

If a child is refusing treatment and they are not Gillick competent, the parents can give consent on behalf of the child. Remember, you must always act in the best interests of the child, so you should consider if overriding the wishes of a distressed child is really necessary. It is better to give the child time and to try to persuade the child that the treatment will help them. A Gillick competent child is legally entitled to refuse to give consent to treatment. In some circumstances refusal can be overridden by those with parental responsibility or by a court of law. The circumstances would be where it is believed that refusing consent to treatment will be detrimental to a child/young person's well-being. Similarly, young people aged 16–17 years can withhold consent to treatment but can be overruled in exceptional circumstances if it is considered to be in their best interests.

When parents withhold consent

If parents withhold consent to treatment and health professionals believe it is not in the child's best interests, legal advice should be sought on how best to proceed.

Activity 7.8 *Decision making*

Fiona is 15 years old and has consented to receiving the human papilloma vaccine (HPV) at school. However, her mother has expressed her disapproval and is refusing to give her consent to Fiona receiving the vaccine. Fiona is a competent young person and has sufficient intelligence and understanding to be fully aware of the nature of the HPV vaccine, its benefits and risks.

- You are the school nurse; should you accept Fiona's consent or follow the wishes of her mother?

An outline answer is provided at the end of the chapter.

Chapter summary

This chapter has discussed how to work effectively in partnership with children/young people and parents/carers. The children's nurse should actively involve children and families in the decision-making process. You should give children and young people explanations of treatments such as medicines that are appropriate to their age and understanding. In order to do this you must learn to communicate effectively with children of all ages, as well as their families and individuals with special needs. We have seen that good record keeping is essential to safe and effective practice, and that the principles are the same regardless of the form in which the records are held.

The law in relation to consent to medical treatment is complex. As a children's nurse you must be clear about the age at which a child or young person is considered capable of consenting for themselves. You have a responsibility to act in the best interests of the child/young person at all times.

Activities: brief outline answers

Activity 7.1 Encouraging parental concordance (page 170)

Ruby and Sally's scenario is not uncommon. Sally cannot see that the steroid is making any difference to Ruby's asthma because she is 'well' when she is giving it. This is what would have been known as 'non-compliance', as Sally has chosen not to follow instructions but to make her own decisions. The aim of care is to work in partnership with Sally and promote concordance. It is important to maintain a rapport with Sally by listening and being non-judgemental. By trying to make Sally feel guilty about Ruby's hospital admission you will just alienate her and make her more reluctant to be open and honest with health professionals in the future. Sally has a right to her own views and decisions about giving medicines to Ruby. Sally is trying to act in Ruby's best interests according to what she knows; however, it seems that she may need further education about asthma and how steroids work in order to make an informed choice. She will need to be fully informed of both the benefits of administering the steroid inhaler and the risks of not giving it. If Sally is made to feel more in control of the decision making and provided with enough information, concordance is more likely to occur.

Activity 7.2 Self-administration (page 171)

- Sophie is an obvious candidate for self-administration as she is very experienced self-administering at home and will continue to do so. She is willing to self-administer and it is likely it will improve her care as she can administer her insulin at regular times to maintain her blood glucose levels. It demonstrates trust in her abilities and promotes her independence, which is good for her psychologically. Taking the responsibility from her during her hospital admission would be disempowering. It is appropriate to supervise her insulin self-administration closely. Her activity levels will have changed with her admission and she will be stressed, and doses may need to be adjusted. Insulin is also a potentially dangerous medicine if not used correctly and there is a need for safe custody. Any bad habits or problems Sophie has with her insulin can be picked up and rectified.

- Jessica is not a candidate for self-administration and will need to have full nurse administration of her medicines. Jessica has a history of paracetamol overdose. Any patient with a recent history of drug or alcohol abuse is not safe for self-administration. Also, Jessica is undergoing a general anaesthetic. Any patient undergoing sedation or general anaesthetic is unsuitable for self-administration. The co-codamol is a new medicine and, while on the ward, full supervision will be required to teach Jessica about the purpose of the medicine, its benefits and side effects, the dosage and how often to take it.

Activity 7.5 Unauthorised access to patient records (page 180)

This is a serious breach of confidentiality; Jane should definitely not be accessing the GP records of her daughter's friend. She has no direct professional relationship with Lucy and is not providing her with nursing care. She is just prying into Lucy's personal information and, if she is found out, the consequences would be serious for her.

Activity 7.6 Parental consent and a 16 year old (page 181)

As Georgia is 16 years old, she is assumed to have the same capacity as an adult to consent to treatment. However, until Georgia is 18 you should encourage her to involve her parents in making such important decisions. If she declines to inform her parents you should abide by her decision.

Activity 7.7 Parental consent and a 14 year old (page 181)

As April is only 14 years of age she would need parental consent for this treatment unless you can establish that she is competent to give consent herself. When considering contraceptive advice or treatment to a person under 16 years without parental consent, we can refer to 'Fraser Guidelines' (DH, 2004b). The nurse or doctor must be satisfied that April will understand the advice; that she cannot be persuaded to tell her parents or allow a health professional to tell her parents that she is seeking contraceptive advice or treatment; that it is likely that April will continue having unprotected sex with or without treatment; and that April may suffer in her physical or mental health unless she receives contraceptive advice or treatment.

Activity 7.8 Parent refusing consent (page 182)

As a competent young person Fiona is entitled to give her consent to treatment. Ideally, her parents would be involved and agree to the treatment, but her mother cannot overrule Fiona's decision. As a school nurse you should have ensured that her mother was properly advised of the benefits and risks of the HPV vaccine. Before administering the vaccine you should be sure that the valid consent form is completed and follow local policy. This could mean completing a 'checklist for competency to consent' form.

Further reading

Bach, S and Grant, A (2009) *Communication and Interpersonal Skills for Nurses.* Exeter: Learning Matters.

This book explores the core concepts of communication and interpersonal skills and is practical and accessible.

Gillick v *West Norfolk and Wisbech AHA* (1986) AC 112 at 113.

This case concerned the rights of children of 16 years or younger to obtain contraception without a parent's permission. You can read it online at **www.hrcr.org/safrica/childrens_rights/Gillick_West Norfolk.htm**.

Griffith, R and Tengnah, C (2008) *Law and Professional Issues in Nursing*, 2nd edition. Exeter: Learning Matters.

Nurses are more accountable than ever to the public, patients, their employers and the profession, and it is vital that they have a clear understanding of legal, ethical and professional issues, as explored in this book.

Royal College of Nursing (RCN) (2006) *Transcultural Healthcare Practice.* London: RCN.

This is an educational resource for nurses and other healthcare professionals and is available online at www.rcn.org.uk/development/learning/transcultural_health/foundation/sectiontwo.

The following three titles are sources of guidance on the difficult topic of consent and are all available through the department's website at **www.dh.gov.uk**:

Department of Health (DH) (2001) *Consent: A Guide for Children and Young People.* London: Department of Health.

Department of Health (DH) (2001) *Consent – What You Have a Right to Expect: A guide for parents.* London: Department of Health.

Department of Health (DH) (2001) *Seeking Consent: Working with children.* London: Department of Health.

Useful websites

www.actionforsickchildren.org

Action for Sick Children is a children's healthcare charity formed to ensure that children always receive the highest standards of care possible. It produces training packs and educational films for healthcare professionals.

www.britishsignlanguage.com

This site uses moving pictures to show the basic signs for British Sign Language.

www.equip.nhs.uk/HealthTopics/languages.aspx

The NHS website Equip provides links to other sites with resources in languages other than English, and to support groups and services for people from ethnic minorities.

www.hpset.org.uk

The Hospital Play Staff Education Trust registers qualified hospital play specialists and sets the qualifying standards.

www.makaton.org

Makaton uses signs and symbols to teach communication, language and literacy skills to people with communication and learning difficulties. There is a wide range of resources to help you learn and use Makaton, produced by the Makaton Charity and by other organisations.

www.nahps.org.uk

The National Association of Hospital Play Staff is a charity that promotes the physical and mental well-being of children and young people in hospitals and hospices or receiving medical care at home. It provides professional support for all hospital play staff.

www.ncb.org.uk/cpis

The Children's Play Information Service is funded by the Department for Culture, Media and Sport, and produces factsheets and student reading on various play topics. It forms part of the National Children's Bureau Library and Information Service.

Chapter 8
Keeping up to date
with evidence-based practice

Chapter aims

By the end of this chapter, you should be able to:

- access commonly used evidence-based sources relating to the safe and effective management of medicine;
- work within national and local policies and ensure others do the same;
- use sources of information, national and local policies and formularies, for example the *British National Formulary* and the *British National Formulary for Children*.

Introduction

All healthcare workers must endeavour to provide the highest standards of care based on the best available evidence of what does and does not work (DH, 1997). Children's nurses are required to provide the best quality care possible to the children and young people in their care. Healthcare decisions are increasingly complex in nature due to the many factors that influence them. In order to make decisions in medicines management and advise parents about treatments, you must use your clinical judgement. Clinical judgements are based on the many sources of evidence available to you. The evidence sources in relation to medicines management include local policies, recommendations, guidelines and the *British National Formulary for Children* (BNFC). However, where there are no local guidelines, you must be able to look further to answer some questions. Other sources of information include national guidance, such as that produced by the National Institute for Health and Clinical Evidence (NICE), or less obvious sources such as expert opinion and peer-reviewed articles. A registered children's nurse needs to have the skills necessary to search for and evaluate the evidence to inform practice.

The Nursing and Midwifery Council *Code*, published in May 2008, states that nurses must provide a high standard of practice and care at all times:

Use the best available evidence

You must deliver care based on the best available evidence or best practice.

You must ensure any advice you give is evidence-based if you are suggesting healthcare products or services.

You must ensure that the use of complementary or alternative therapies is safe and in the best interests of those in your care.

What is evidence-based practice?

It is now considered unacceptable that patients requiring healthcare can receive care that is not based on best practice. Evidence-based practice is an approach to patient care that encourages healthcare providers to consider and synthesise the best available evidence. The evidence available includes empirical research, expert opinion, and patient values and expectations. Sound evidence should be an integral part of clinical decision making. For example, let us consider the management of babies with colic. Historically, colic has been treated for hundreds of years using traditional remedies such as gripe water, fennel oil and chamomile tea. However, the evidence for the effectiveness of these treatments has been from anecdotal accounts and there is much speculation about their use. Anecdotal evidence is at the bottom of the hierarchy of evidence in healthcare practice. More recently, it has been suggested that treatments such as cranial osteopathy, probiotics, simeticone and lactase are effective treatments. In fact, no treatment has been shown to be of any considerable benefit for infantile colic. There have been many research studies conducted of interventions for infantile colic, but most have been of a poor methodological quality. It is often confusing for nurses as to what is the best advice to give to parents.

We can see a shift in healthcare culture away from basing our decisions on what was traditionally accepted practice and opinion, towards making use of research and sound evidence to guide clinical decisions. For nurses to follow evidence-based practice (Figure 8.1) and make sense of the evidence, they need first to be able to turn problems into a focused clinical question. You must be able to systematically search for literature to address your questions, appraise the literature for its usefulness and validity, and apply your findings to your practice (Sackett et al., 1997).

What is research?

Research is the activity of searching for knowledge, discovering new things and increasing our understanding. In healthcare research there is a diverse range of activities, from discovering how to improve treatments, to uncovering adverse effects of medicines or lifestyles. Healthcare research is a systematic approach to gathering information in order to answer a question. Before

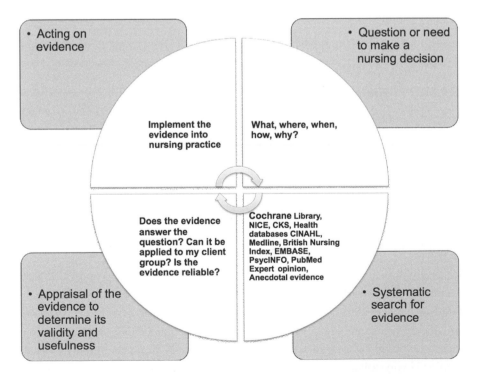

Figure 8.1: Evidence-based practice

any research takes place, the researcher must be clear about the purpose of the study. The fundamental areas of activity to which research is central are description, explanation, evidence gathering and generalisation. The type of research activity chosen will depend on the type of question the researcher is trying to answer. Research cannot give a definite answer but simply collects the best evidence available at the time. Research methodology is full of problems and often future research will overturn the findings.

Types of research studies

Research is a broad term covering a range of different types of study, each with a different design. The different studies will present you with different types of evidence that range from the anecdotal to the more scientific evidence obtained from controlled clinical trials. In healthcare research there are two types of research studies called **quantitative** and **qualitative.** Quantitative research tends to be associated with scientific enquiry and viewing the world in a measurable way. Quantitative research often starts with a **hypothesis** to be tested and uses established research methods. Qualitative research is used to gain understanding of how people feel and their motivations, attitudes, behaviours and value systems. The use of a quantitative or qualitative method of enquiry would depend on the nature of the question being asked (see Table 8.1).

Purpose of research	**Types of research study**	**Example**
To describe an existing situation	Descriptive studies (surveys of practice and patients)	What are the wound dressing choices of children's nurses?
To look for explanations for existing behaviour	Qualitative research studies (interviews/surveys)	Perceptions and concerns of being a student nurse
To test a hypothesis based on a prediction	Quantitative research studies (clinical trials)	Ametop gel is more effective than Emla cream for local anesthesia
To seek out generalisations	Systematic reviews of controlled trials	Cochrane Reviews – antibiotics for whooping cough

Table 8.1: Examples of research activity

Within healthcare there is a typical hierarchy of evidence when considering evidence-based practice (Oxford Centre for Evidence-based Medicine, 2009). The hierarchy provides you with a framework to review the available evidence and make a clinical judgement (see Figure 8.2). When evaluating research the hierarchy should be used as a guide, rather than a set of inflexible rules. You must take into consideration other factors, such as the population studied and the quality of the research, before deciding if you can apply the evidence to your practice. Regardless of the research method used, if the quality of the study was poor, you must regard the findings with suspicion.

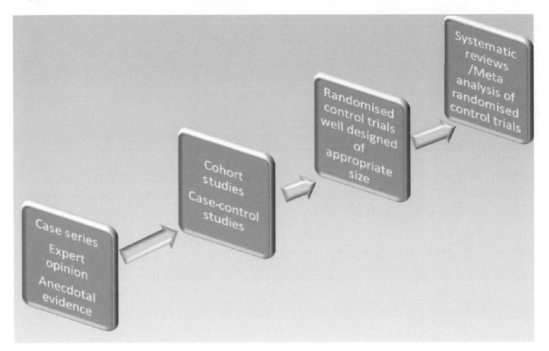

Figure 8.2: Hierarchy of evidence

Systematic reviews

Systematic reviews are an evaluation of the existing research evidence relevant to a given question. Often one clinical trial by itself has limited information. A systematic review brings together all the controlled trials of a research question in order to synthesise the information and then evaluate the findings over a range of patient groups.

Meta-analysis

Meta-analysis is a statistical technique that can combine the findings of two or more clinical trials. Well-conducted meta-analysis allows for a more objective appraisal of the effectiveness of health-care interventions.

Randomised controlled trials

Randomised controlled (or control) trials (RCTs) are a form of experimental research in which the subjects are randomly allocated into two groups. One group (experimental group) receives the intervention or treatment being tested, and the other group (the control group) receives a placebo or alternative treatment. The results of the trial are assessed by comparing the experimental group with the control group. Randomised controlled trials are the 'gold standard' for assessing the effectiveness of an intervention. They are the most rigorous way to determine a cause and effect relationship between a treatment and outcome.

Cohort studies

Cohort studies involve observing a group (cohort) of subjects over a period of time. They can be prospective studies, which follow the subjects into the future, or retrospective studies, which look at information from the subject's past.

Case-control studies

A case-control study is a comparison of a group of people who have a condition with a group who do not.

Case reports and case series

A case report is a detailed record of a single individual (case report) or small group (case series) response to a treatment or specific environmental exposure. They are useful sources of evidence when a treatment or illness is very rare or for new medications or off-label use of medications.

Concept summary

The following hypothetical scenario illustrates the differences between the types of research studies.

A mother notices that her young son has extraordinary night vision and is convinced that it is due to the fact that she fed him carrot juice every day. She recommends carrot juice to her friends for their babies. This story is an **anecdote**. Although the anecdote may be plausible, it doesn't prove anything. The local health visitor is quite interested in this idea, and decides to advise some local mothers to feed their babies carrot juice, which results in a number of **case reports**. When she has a small group of case reports she produces a **case series**. This is slightly more convincing than an anecdote on the hierarchy of evidence. The community pediatrician decides that the case series should be more rigidly defined and decides to undertake a **cohort study**. The cohort study includes a group of children within a specific age range who are given a precise amount of carrot juice every day. In this way, the group of children can be followed over a period of time after the course of carrot juice to see if they develop extraordinary night vision. Some conclusions of the effects of the carrot juice and the night vision may be drawn, but any changes in the night vision could be due to other factors (e.g. the extraordinary night vision may be due to other foods the children are eating). A **clinical trial** is necessary in order to discover the specific effects of carrot juice above all other factors. In the clinical trial there is a treatment group (who receive carrot juice) and a control group who do everything the same as the treatment group apart from the fact that they receive no carrot juice. The most superior form of a clinical trial is a **randomised controlled trial**, in which the children are randomly allocated to groups (to avoid bias) and the experimenters are blinded. 'Blinded' means that the experimenter does not know which child is in the control group or the treatment group (to avoid bias). Double-blinded is when the child/parent does not know if they are receiving

continued overleaf . . .

continued . . .
carrot juice or a placebo (to avoid bias). To get a more convincing result of the true effect, the results of a number of RCTs are synthesised together in a **systematic review**.

Note that, although carrots are high in vitamin A and do help maintain healthy eyesight, the night vision rumour was British propaganda during the Second World War to distract the Germans from discovering that the British were using radar!

Factors affecting the reliability of research studies

When reviewing the evidence you must be aware that there are many factors that affect how reliable the research study is. Outcome measures must be valid and sensitive. How do we define and measure what extraordinary eyesight is, for example? How do we know how much carrot juice is needed to result in extraordinary eyesight? What if we gave them too little, or too much? The number of children in the study must be large enough; too small a group runs the risk that the true effect of the treatment or intervention will be lost. (How many children need to be fed carrot juice to give a convincing result?) There are statistical formulas for calculating the optimum sample sizes that must be followed for the study to be reliable. In general, the less effective the treatment, the larger the sample size will need to be to discover a difference between the control group and treatment group.

Clinical trials need to have a group of untreated controls against which the patients in the treatment group can be compared. This is because some conditions can just get better by themselves without treatment. For example, the children being treated with carrot juice could have developed extraordinary eyesight because the government had banned TV viewing. The group treated with carrot juice could be compared to the control group to see if findings where similar. RCTs are very difficult to perform and do not always go to plan, which can limit their usefulness. The response and behaviour of participants in a research study are influenced by what they know and believe. In research there is a particular risk of that belief influencing findings. This is more likely to happen when there is an element of subjectivity in the assessment, which would lead to a bias result. For this reason 'blinding' is used to eliminate the bias. This means that the study participants are kept unaware of their assigned treatment. Double-blinding keeps the researchers who are involved in the allocation of treatment, data collection and analysing of the results unaware also, so they are not influenced by that awareness. Blinding can fail, however; for example, it is very hard for the mothers not to notice if it is carrot juice they are feeding their children.

Giving the control group an orange-coloured drink and telling them it is carrot juice is called using a placebo. This intervention can lead the parent and child to believe that the drink will make their eyesight better and produce a subjective perception of extraordinary eyesight. This is known as the placebo effect. Only when the carrot juice shows an effect on eyesight over and above the placebo effect is it considered to be efficacious for extraordinary eyesight.

There are many other problems and flaws that will limit what conclusion can be drawn. Patients can be lost to follow up, or may decide not to continue. It is sometimes hard to be sure if they stuck to the treatment. How likely is it that the children would drink that carrot juice or placebo every day? Perhaps they would exaggerate the truth so as not to disappoint you?

No study is perfect and one trial alone is rarely conclusive.

Critiquing frameworks

Critical appraisal is a skill that is essential to providing evidence-based nursing care. There are several critiquing frameworks within the nursing literature to help you evaluate research studies. The NHS Critical Appraisal Skills Programme has developed a number of tools to help individuals with the critical appraisal of different types of research, and these are free to download (see 'Useful websites' at the end of the chapter).

Parent/child preference

Having a rigid view of evidence-based practice means that we accept only practice that is underpinned by sound research evidence. Research evidence is not always available to support or disprove the effectiveness of all treatments, in particular those clinical presentations that are complex and varied. In the example of the treatments for infantile colic, we cannot rely on the research evidence as it was of poor methodological quality. The treatments are not proven to be effective, but are not disproven. Perhaps we should use McKibbon and Walker's (1994) less rigid definition of evidence based practice: *An approach to healthcare that promotes the collection, interpretation and integration of valid, important and applicable patient reported, clinician observed, and research derived evidence.*

When we are considering applying current best evidence to individual patients, we should consider all the dimensions of that individual and the outcomes of the treatment or intervention. We should respect the right of the parent or child/young person to choose their own treatment and care from all the available options. Evidenced-based practice should focus on avoiding harm and placing the child's interests above all others.

> ## Scenario
>
> *Seventeen-year-old Jade has been using Infacol drops for the treatment of her 4-week-old baby's colic and has found it to be really effective. She asks if she can have a prescription from the doctor for the Infacol as she finds it too expensive to buy it herself.*
>
> • *After reading the Clinical Knowledge Summary (see Activity 8.1 on page 195) on the management of infantile colic, should you encourage the continued use and prescribing of Infacol?*

You would be wrong now to believe that all practice should be based entirely on research. Although there is no strong research evidence that Infacol (simeticone) is effective, we cannot be certain that, for Jade's baby, it is not having a positive outcome. Jade's personal evidence justifies the continued use. In this specific situation Jade feels a benefit and, as far as she is concerned, the

Infacol is doing what it is intended to do and improving the colic. The treatment is having the desired effect on patient outcomes, and Jade is happy. The cost of the treatment is relatively inexpensive to achieve the desired outcome, and the treatment is considered to be doing no harm. Withdrawal of the treatment could lead to a return of the colic, parental stress and the use of less desirable alternatives.

Until empirical research evidence is available, healthcare providers must provide evidence-based practice that balances the most current research evidence with clinical expertise and the preferences of the child/young person and parent/carer. Achieving this balance is often difficult, remembering that you must always remain professionally accountable for your actions and provide cost-effective care. The evidence exists to inform and guide practice rather than dictate practice. (See Figure 8.3.)

How can you ensure best evidence is used in practice?

To ensure that best evidence is used in practice you must be motivated to deliver evidence-based practice. This means finding the best evidence with which to answer the questions that arise in

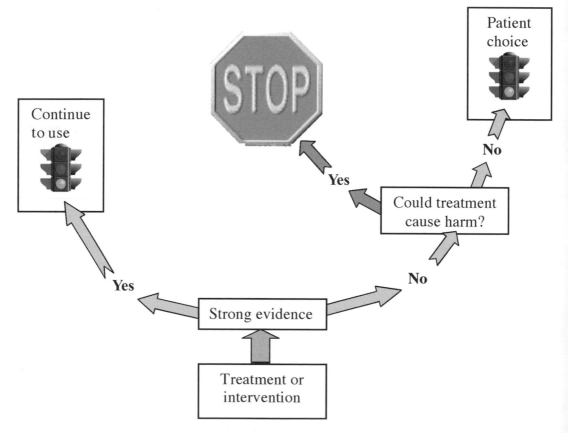

Figure 8.3: Road map of evidence-based practice

practice. You must learn to appraise the evidence critically and apply the results to the practice decisions.

Where is the evidence?

The NHS and other organisations provide an expanding range of information resources for evidence-based practice. They are designed to help busy practitioners to access reliable information to inform their practice decisions. The NHS Clinical Knowledge Summaries provide evidence-based information about common conditions managed in primary care.

Activity 8.1   *Evidence-based practice and research*

Go to the NHS Clinical Knowledge Summaries (CKS) website by either using Google or going to **www.cks.nhs.uk/home**. Search in the topics section or alphabetically for 'infantile colic'.

- What is the suggested advice to give to parents about infantile colic?

An outline answer is provided at the end of the chapter.

NHS Evidence is a health information electronic resource (formerly the National Library for Health). Resources the website provides include evidence-based reviews, NICE guidelines, e-books and journals. The available healthcare databases include **AMED**, **MEDLINE**, **British Nursing Index**, **CINAHL**, **EMBASE**, **HMIC**, **PsycINFO**, **PubMed** and **ZETOC**. The major healthcare databases contain all kinds of research as well as non-research materials such as comments and editorials. The healthcare databases enable you to search the available research evidence in order to answer specific clinical questions. The NHS Evidence website also includes access to *British National Formulary for Children* and the National Electronic Library for Medicines. The website is freely available to NHS employees through Athens registration, including student nurses.

Evidence-based practice in medicines management

Medicines management includes the selection, acquisition, storage, prescribing, administration and evaluation of effectiveness of medicines. Evidence-based practice in medicines management is the use of the best evidence available in relation to these areas. It requires that you regularly review and question your reasons for using certain treatments. This is because new evidence becomes available all the time through research or audit that may suggest that another treatment is preferable. Other reasons might be that preparations are unavailable or discontinued or have become too expensive compared to other treatment options. Specific patient circumstances may be an allergic response to, or intolerance or dislike of, the preferred treatment option, which will require you to find a suitable alternative.

When a question arises, you must search for and appraise the evidence available and then implement a clinical decision, taking into consideration the patient's perspective. For example, if we consider wound care and medicines management, the choice of a suitable dressing will need to take into account the type of wound, the dressings available, the patient's individual circumstances and choice, the cost and evidence of effectiveness. There are many wound dressings available for you to choose from, so how do you decide on what is best?

Scenario

You are a community children's nurse and are looking after 4-year-old Lizzie, who has a minor burn on her arm. How do you decide which dressing to use on the burn? How do you ensure that you are providing evidence-based practice and good medicines management?

You need to ask a series of questions in order to make a clinical decision on what dressing to use. First, what evidence is there of the use of different wound dressings in the management of minor burns in children?

To answer this question you would need to search the healthcare databases for the best evidence available. There is little evidence or consensus on the most appropriate dressing for minor burns. The NHS Clinical Knowledge Summary advice for the management of superficial dermal burns is to use a non-adherent dressing, such as paraffin gauze, silicone-coated nylon dressing, polyurethane film or hydrocolloid dressing. In clean, partial-thickness burns, dressing with paraffin-impregnated gauze (Jelonet) is generally preferred. Jelonet is cheap and in plentiful supply. As long as it is applied in multiple layers to prevent drying out, which can result in it sticking to the wound, there is little evidence to suggest that any other form of dressing improves results.

There is no specific advice given for children. Gotschall et al. (1998) found that wounds treated with Mepitel healed significantly faster and patients experienced less pain when compared to treatment with Flamazine in the management of partial-thickness scald wounds in children. It was uncertain as to whether the faster healing time was related to the effect of silicone on epithelial growth or to a decrease in cell damage compared to the Flamazine group. The study recommended a larger-scale trial to confirm the results. A Cochrane Review (Wasiak et al., 2008) summarised the literature on methods of treating partial-thickness burns. The Review found the literature for each dressing type to be limited due to quantity and methodological quality.

There is insufficient evidence to recommend a particular type of dressing for partial-thickness burns. There is limited evidence to support the use of hydrocolloids (e.g. DuoDerm), polyurethane films (e.g. Tegaderm), hydrogels (e.g. Curagel), silicone-coated nylon (e.g. Mepitel), biosynthetic skin substitutes (e.g. Biobrane), silver-impregnated dressings (e.g. Acticoat) and hydrofiber (e.g. Aquacel). All the dressings proved to be superior to the use of silver sulfadiazine (e.g. Flamazine) and the practice of routinely treating partial-thickness burns with it should be re-examined.

How does the above evidence help you to select a wound dressing?

The evidence does not give you a clear indication of which wound care product you should use for a partial-thickness burn. It does indicate that you should not routinely use Flamazine. The NHS Clinical Knowledge Summary advises use of a non-adherent dressing – Jelonet is generally preferred.

You should now ask the following questions.

- Are there local policies or clinical guidelines for the management of a minor burn in children?
- Who are the experts in this area and what is the expert opinion?
- Does the parent/child have a particular preference?
- How frequently does the dressing need to be changed compared to other dressings?
- Do I need specific training to use this dressing?
- Are there any contraindications for use with this patient?
- Is it suitable for use in children?
- What is the cost of the preferred dressing compared to the others? Is it more cost effective to use a more expensive dressing that requires less frequent changes?
- Are there any specific storage requirements? What is the shelf life of the product?
- Is the preferred dressing available on prescription?

You will base your decision on the answers to the above questions and your interpretation of the evidence.

Wound care products are classified as a medical device (MHRA, 2008) and are approved as safe and fit for purpose by UK Notified Bodies appointed by the MHRA. They have not had to undergo rigorous clinical trials like medicines. No product is completely safe and will have side effects, which may be very minor or possibly quite serious. A healthcare professional who uses as device such as a wound dressing against the manufacturer's instructions or in a way it is not intended is liable for any consequences.

How will you review the clinical effectiveness of the dressing you have chosen?

Clinical effectiveness is an important aspect of evidence-based practice. As a nurse you have a responsibility to ensure that you do not waste time, effort and resources on treatments that have no therapeutic advantage (Alderson and Groves, 2004). There will be many circumstances when you will find that the evidence is not clear or is conflicting. In order to practise safely as a registered nurse you will need to be knowledgeable of the sources of evidence that will help inform your clinical decision making. These sources include Cochrane Reviews, Clinical Knowledge Summaries, local guidelines, journal articles and expert opinion.

Costs of evidence-based medicines management

A report by the Audit Commission, *A Spoonful of Sugar* (2001), on the use of medicines in NHS hospitals found that medicine use is not always optimised, which leads to poorer-quality care and higher costs. The report found that medication errors occur far too often and their effects on patients and the cost to the NHS is substantial. Financial consideration should be central to all decisions made by healthcare staff in relation to medicines management within the NHS. Decisions on the choice of medicines or treatment should be based on the best available evidence, patient preference and cost.

> ### Scenario
>
> *You are working on a surgical day case ward where all paediatric surgical patients have EMLA cream applied to both hands prior to cannulation and anaesthetic induction.*
>
> * *Consider why the department routinely uses EMLA cream. What would be a good argument for using Ametop gel as an alternative?*

Some departments routinely use EMLA cream as a topical anaesthetic prior to venepuncture and cannulation in children, whereas others use Ametop. It is important to consider and question the reasons for this rather than accepting what is traditionally used.

* **Efficacy**. Studies seem to suggest that Ametop gel has better anaesthetic effect than EMLA cream (Arrowsmith and Campbell, 2000; Choy et al., 1999; Lawson et al., 1995; Romsing et al., 1999; Van Kam et al., 1997). Ametop gel has the advantage of a faster onset of topical anaesthesia (30 minutes for venepuncture; 45 minutes for cannulation) than EMLA, which should be applied 1 hour before the procedure. Another advantage to Ametop gel is its increased vasodilating properties. Adverse effects in comparison to EMLA are similar.
* **Cost**. The use of Ametop could also produce a potential cost saving. The unit cost of Ametop is less than that of EMLA cream.

It would seem that Ametop gel is preferable to the use of EMLA cream based on the present evidence as well as the potential cost savings. Healthcare workers must question their existing practice in order to improve the quality of patient care and reduce the costs of medicines.

Research and medicines used in children

At present, many of the medicines and treatments used in children have only been tested in adults. This means that there are fewer medicines available for children to take and we know a lot less about how drugs work in young children. Any new medicine must be properly tested through clinical trials before it is approved for use. The clinical trials are designed to tell us whether the medicine works better than current treatments, if it is safe, whether there are side effects and what doses work best.

Limited numbers of clinical trials have been conducted with children, mainly due to ethical or commercial reasons. The result of the limited research has meant that many medicines used in children are off-label or unlicensed. This means that children are exposed to adult preparations and are at greater risk of adverse reactions. It is important that clinical trials are carried out on children as well as adults, as children are very different and the effects may not be the same. Children will then benefit from more child-friendly medicines that are safer for them to use. A new regulation to improve the health of children in Europe was adopted by the European Parliament in 2006. Part of the objective of Regulation EC No 1901/2006 is to increase high-quality ethical research into medicines for children.

Medical research may focus on scientific experimentation with drug regimes and protocols to establish those that are most effective, and children's nurses may at times be asked to assist in medical research. Children's nurses are responsible for the delivery of drugs to patients and the assessment of their effects, and have an important role in the assessment and evaluation of medicines used and ensuring patient safety and informed consent. Clinical research nursing is a specialist role focused on the care of research participants and includes implementing protocols, data collection, recording and patient follow-up.

Nurses should also have their own research agenda in order to broaden their knowledge base in relation to medicines management. Research is an essential part of informing child nursing practice and helping to establish a professional practice base for medicines management. The aim of nursing research is to improve practice and maintain high standards in all areas related to medicines. This may include such areas of practice as parental and child/young person knowledge and attitudes towards medicine use, parental and child adherence, or teaching strategies. Nursing research into the quality of care in medicines administration enables us to identify ineffective and unsafe practices and discontinue them.

Evidence-based practice and CAMs

Complementary and alternative medicines (CAMs) include various therapies and disciplines that are health-related but not considered to be conventional medicines. The use of CAMs is common in child healthcare in the UK. Many nurses are choosing to practise such therapies as baby massage, aromatherapy and reflexology. Parents are choosing to access and use cranial osteopathy, acupuncture, homeopathy and herbal medicines. This raises the question as to whether research has been carried out and whether there are adequate information sources to make clinical decisions. The ethos of evidence-based practice should extend to CAMs (House of Lords, 2000). Registered nurses are often asked by patients to help them to gain information on CAMs and nurses are obliged to help patients exercise their choices. It is advisable for you to encourage patients to direct some of their questions towards those offering the complementary therapies.

When considering a CAM therapy, you will need to find out if evidence is available and how it can inform practice. You must decide if the research used a suitable methodology and if it can be applied to child healthcare practice. If there is only anecdotal evidence available, how will it affect your decision making? You must never practise without adequate training and supervision within this area. The RCN has produced guidance for nurses who wish to integrate complementary therapies into clinical care (RCN, 2003).

Scenario

Laura is struggling to cope with her 2-year-old daughter Olivia's eczema. She has a friend who says that her eczema was 'cured' by using Chinese herbal medicine and Laura is quite interested in trying it for Olivia. She feels she has nothing to lose and has already enquired about seeing a local Chinese herbalist. You are a community children's nurse caring for Olivia, and Laura would like your advice.

This is not an uncommon scenario and one that you should be prepared for. If you search the evidence, you will find that the National Collaborating Centre for Women's and Children's Health (2007) has produced clinical guidelines for the management of atopic eczema in children. The guidelines state that the effectiveness and safety of complementary therapies such as herbal medicine have not been adequately assessed in clinical studies. You should inform Laura that she should be wary of using herbal medicines with Olivia, particularly any medicine that does not have clear instructions in English on its safe usage. Laura should be made aware that topical corticosteroids have been known to have been intentionally added to some herbal products for use in children with atopic eczema, and that liver toxicity has been related to some Chinese herbal medicines for atopic eczema. Laura should inform her healthcare professionals if she is using any herbal therapies and continue to use emollients on Olivia's skin. You should advise Laura that regular massage with emollients may improve Olivia's atopic eczema.

Chapter summary

This chapter has defined what evidence-based practice means and how it affects you as a nurse. You should now be aware that you must deliver nursing care that is based on the best available evidence or best practice. Any advice you give and the use of complementary or alternative therapies should be evidence-based. To ensure best evidence is used in practice, you must learn to turn your problems into questions and search for the evidence in order to appraise it and apply the results to your practice decisions. We have established that research is the activity of searching for knowledge and discovering new things to increase our understanding. There are many different types of studies and the hierarchy of evidence and critiquing frameworks can be used as a guide when evaluating the available research. There are numerous healthcare databases that enable you to search the available evidence and they are available free to NHS employees through Athens registration. This chapter has identified that research evidence is not always available to answer all the questions that arise in practice, in particular those questions that are multifaceted. When applying evidenced-based practice to individual patients we must consider a less rigid approach that takes into consideration the patient's choices as well as the research-derived evidence.

Activities: brief outline answers

Activity 8.1 Researching infantile colic (page 195)

The NHS Clinical Knowledge home page is easy to find using the Google search engine. You can search under the topic 'child health' or by alphabet by clicking in the left-hand browser.

The suggested advice to give to parents for the management of infantile colic is all non-pharmacological.

- *Reassure the parents that their baby is well, they are not doing something wrong, the baby is not rejecting them, and that colic is common and is a phase that will pass within a few months.*
- *Holding the baby through the crying episode may be helpful. However, if there are times when the crying feels intolerable, it is best to put the baby down somewhere safe (e.g. their cot) and take a few minutes' 'time out'.*

- *Other strategies that may help to soothe a crying infant include:*
  - *Gentle motion (e.g. pushing the pram or a ride in the car).*
  - *'White noise' (e.g. vacuum cleaner, hairdryer, running water).*
  - *Bathing in a warm bath.*
- *Encourage parents to look after their own well-being:*
  - *Ask family and friends for support – parents need to be able to take a break.*
  - *Rest when the baby is asleep.*
  - *Meet other parents with babies of the same age.*

(www.cks.nhs.uk/home)

Remember that good medicines management sometimes means not advising the use of medicines. If you read the full CK Summary you will find the information you need to give to parents and make a clinical decision on other treatments such as simeticone and lactase drops.

Further reading

McKenna, H, Cutliffe, J and McKenna, P (1999) Evidence-based practice: demolishing some myths. *Nursing Standard*, 14(16): 39–42.

This article examines alternatives to evidence-based practice, and is available at **www.clinical governance.scot.nhs.uk/documents/v14w16p3942.pdf**.

Sackett, DL, Rosenberg, WMC, Gray, JAM and Richardson, WS (1996). Evidence based medicine: what it is and what it isn't. *British Medical Journal*, 312 (13 January): 71–2.

This article is about integrating individual clinical expertise and the best evidence from elsewhere. The full text is available via an Athens account at **www.bmj/content/312/7023/71.extract**.

Useful websites

www.cks.nhs.uk/home

The NHS Clinical Knowledge Summaries are aimed at healthcare professionals working in primary care and are a reliable source of evidence-based information.

www.library.nhs.uk/default.aspx

NHS Evidence is a Health Information Resource (formerly the National Library for Health).

http://metalib.kcl.ac.uk

This url will take you to ISS Electronic resources, a King's College London site that provides a list of evidence-based practice electronic resources and databases.

www.mhra.gov.uk/index.htm

The Medicines and Healthcare products Regulatory Agency safeguards the public by regulating medicines and devices. This site provides guidance, safety information, warnings and reports on medicines and medical devices.

www.nice.org.uk

The National Institute for Health and Clinical Evidence is an independent organisation responsible for providing national guidance on promoting good health and preventing and treating ill health.

www.npc.co.uk

The National Prescribing Centre supports the NHS and its staff to improve quality, safety and value for money in the use of medicines. There is a merger planned with NICE in April 2011.

www.npsa.nhs.uk

The National Patient Safety Agency informs and influences the health sector in order to improve patient safety and care.

www.sph.nhs.uk/what-we-do/public-health-workforce/resources/critical-appraisals-skills-programme

The NHS Critical Appraisal Skills Programme (CASP) aims to help individuals to develop skills and make sense of research evidence. Critical appraisal tools are available free to download for personal use.

www.thecochranelibrary.com/view/0/index.html

The Cochrane Library is a collection of databases that contain different types of high-quality evidence to inform healthcare decision making.

Glossary

AMED: the Allied and Complementary Medicine Database, a bibliographic database produced by the Health Care Information Service of the British Library. It covers a selection of journals in complementary medicine, palliative care and several professions allied to medicine.

Ampoule: a glass container for liquid medicine for injection.

Anecdotal evidence: a personal account of an event, which is not necessarily true.

Apnoea monitor: a breathing monitor with sensors that set off an alarm if a baby or child stops breathing.

Aqueous solution: a solution that is dissolved in water or is similar to water.

Bilirubin: bile pigment that is the product of the breakdown of haemoglobin in the liver.

British Nursing Index: a bibliographic database that indexes articles from the most popular English language nursing journals published primarily in the UK.

Capsule: a medicine enclosed in a hard or soft shell.

Carbamazapine: a drug used for the treatment of epilepsy.

Carcinogenic: capable of causing cancer.

Case report: a detailed report of the symptoms, signs, diagnosis, treatment, progress and follow-up of an individual patient.

Case series: a research study that tracks a number of patients with the same intervention or exposure who are given similar treatment.

Caution: a specific warning to be careful, especially with medicine.

Chief Pharmacist: a healthcare professional who is responsible for managing pharmacy services and operations for the local area.

CINAHL: a database covering all aspects of nursing and allied health disciplines.

Clinical trial: a study that follows selected individuals, some receiving a medical intervention (e.g. a drug) and some not.

Cohort study: a study following a predetermined group of individuals through time and measuring the incidence of predetermined outcomes.

Concordance: describes a partnership approach to prescribing and taking medicine. It is different from *compliance*, which describes the patient taking a medicine in relation to the prescriber's instructions.

Cream: semi-solid emulsion that is a mixture of oils and water. Oil-in-water creams are composed of small droplets of oil dispersed in a water base, and water-in-oil creams are small droplets of water dissolved in an oily base.

Cushing's syndrome: a hormone disorder caused by high levels of cortisol in the blood. This can be caused by taking glucocorticoid drugs, or by some types of tumour.

Cytotoxic: describes a drug that prevents cell division.

Denaturation: a structural change in a drug caused by extreme conditions.

Digoxin: a drug used for the treatment of heart conditions.

Diluents: a substance that dilutes another substance.

Efficacy: effectiveness in producing the intended result.

Elixir: a clear, sweet-flavoured liquid that contains alcohol, water and medicine.

EMBASE: a major biomedical and pharmaceutical database indexing thousands of international journals.

Emollient: a hydrating agent composed of fat or oil and applied topically to soften skin.

Enteric coated: refers to tablets or capsules with a coating to prevent their breakdown in the stomach. The contents of coated tablets or capsules will be released only when the dose reaches the intestine. This may be done to protect the drug from stomach acid, to protect the stomach from drug irritation, or to delay the onset of action of the drug.

Epithelial: refers to the layer of cells lining the intestine and through which nutrients are absorbed.

Extended formulary nurse prescribing: a type of independent nurse prescribing where nurses were able to prescribe from a limited range of medicines for specific conditions. It was introduced in 2002 for four therapeutic areas: minor ailments, minor injuries, health promotion and palliative care. Amendments to legislation in 2006 to enable nurse independent prescribers to prescribe any licensed medicine for any medical condition within their competence, including some controlled drugs, replaced the need for extended formulary prescribing.

Extravasation: passage or escape into the tissues.

Gillick competent: a term used in law that refers to a child under the age of 16 years having the capacity to consent to their own medical treatment, without the need for their parents to give permission or be informed.

Hepatic microsomal enzyme system: a group of enzymes associated with the liver that play a role in the metabolism of many drugs.

HMIC: the Health Management Information Consortium database is a compilation of data from two sources: the Department of Health's Library and Information Services, and King's Fund Information and Library Service.

Hypothesis: an idea that quantitative research sets out to prove.

Infiltration: the diffusion of substances into tissue or fat not normal to it or in amounts in excess of the normal.

Invaginate: to push the wall of a cavity into itself.

Ionisation: the separation of molecules into electrically charged atoms.

Kernicterus: damage to the brain of infants caused by increased levels of unconjugated bilirubin.

Licensed use: the indication, age group, dose and route of administration for which a particular drug is authorised to be used by the licensing authority, the Medicines Control Agency. Pharmaceutical companies cannot promote an unlicensed product or a licensed product for an unlicensed indication.

Lipid based: describes a biological compound that is not soluble in water, e.g. a fat, triglyceride, phospholipid or oil.

Loading dose: an initial higher dose of a drug that may be given at the beginning of a course of treatment before dropping down to a lower maintenance dose. It is given in order to quickly achieve therapeutic levels in the blood.

Lumen: the central space within the gastrointestinal tract.

Maintenance dose: the quantity of drug necessary to continue producing a desired effect.

Maintenance fluid: the amount of fluid needed to replace the insensible losses (from breathing, through the skin, and in the stool).

Medicine trail: the path taken by medicines from manufacturers or other suppliers to the wards via the pharmacy. At each point of the trail proper procedures are recommended to ensure that there is adequate record keeping, ensuring the security of medicines.

Medicines Management Committee: this consists of doctors, pharmacists and representatives of other key decision makers in the use of medicines in primary and secondary care. The function of the committee is to review selected pharmaceutical products to assess their clinical value, safety and suitability for use.

MEDLINE: the United States National Library of Medicine's bibliographic database, which provides information from medicine, nursing and allied health.

Modified release: describes a tablet or capsule that has been adapted in some way so that the drug is released slowly. This means that the medicine does not have to be taken too often, which can therefore improve patient compliance. Modifying the release also means that there are smaller peaks and troughs in blood levels and increases the likelihood of therapeutic effectiveness for a longer period of time.

Mole: a unit that refers to the number of particles in a substance.

Molarity of a solution: refers to the number of moles of solute dissolved in one litre of solution.

Molar solution: a mixture of one or more substances (solutes) dispersed molecularly in a sufficient quantity of a dissolving medium (solvent).

Mutagenic: describes something that increases the mutation of DNA in cells.

Occlusion: a closure or blockage.

Ointment: an oil-based medical preparation that is applied topically.

Oxygen saturation monitor: a device that monitors the oxygen saturation of a patient's blood by placing a probe on the skin.

Parenteral: describes drug administration other than by mouth or rectum (enteral), such as injection or infusion.

Perfusion: the circulation of blood through a blood vessel or other channel within the body.

pH: a measure of how acid or alkaline a substance is.

Phenytoin: a drug used for the treatment of epilepsy.

Phlebitis: inflammation of the wall of a vein.

Prescriber: a person in healthcare who is permitted by law to order the use of drugs that legally require a prescription.

Prescription: a written order, issued by a qualified practitioner, that authorises a chemist to supply a specific medication to a patient.

Prodrug: a drug that is administered to the patient in an inactive form and becomes active only after it is metabolised in the body into an active form. The rationale for the use of a prodrug is to optimise absorption, distribution, metabolism and excretion.

Product labels: all medicines in the UK have approved product labels, which must include detailed information on the medicine and how it should be used.

PsycINFO: a database that provides extensive international coverage of the literature on psychology and allied fields.

PubMed: a service of the US National Library of Medicine that includes over 17 million citations from MEDLINE and other life science journals for biomedical articles dating back to the 1950s.

Qualitative: a type of research that seeks to understand the quality or character of human experience and behaviour. It generates non-numerical data such as a child's description of their pain rather than a measure of pain.

Quantitative: a type of systematic research that generates numerical data or data that can be converted into numbers, for example clinical trials.

Randomised controlled trial: a quantitative research study in which patients are allocated randomly (by chance alone) into an intervention group or a control group. The control group may receive standard practice or a placebo or no intervention at all. The trial compares the outcomes of the control group and the intervention group.

Side effects: the unwanted effects of a drug.

Soluble: able to be dissolved in another substance.

Stratum corneum: the outermost layer of the epidermis (the outer layer of skin).

Suppository: a solid bullet-shaped medicine designed to be inserted into the rectum, where it melts at body temperature and is absorbed into the blood vessels in the surrounding tissue.

Suspension: a dispersion of particles in a liquid.

Sustained release: an oral medicine such as a tablet that is designed to be absorbed at various levels in the gastrointestinal tract, therefore prolonging the action.

Systematic review: a review that tries to identify, appraise and synthesise all the high-quality research evidence relevant to a research question.

Teratogenic: refers to a substance that will adversely affect the normal development of a foetus.

Therapeutic index: the ratio between a therapeutic dose of a drug and a toxic dose.

Vesicle: a small sac containing fluid.

ZETOC: a database providing access to the British Library's Electronic Table of Contents of around 20,000 current journals.

References

Alderson, P and Groves, T (2004) What doesn't work and how to show it? *British Medical Journal*, 328: 473.

Allen, K, Golden, LH and Izzo, JL et al. (2001) Normalization of hypertensive responses during ambulatory surgical stress by perioperative music. *Psychosomatic Medicine*, 63 (May/June): 487–92.

American Academy of Pediatrics (AAP), Committee on Drugs (1997) Alternative routes of drug administration: advantages and disadvantages (subject review) (1995–97). *Pediatrics*, 100(1) (July): 143–52.

Arrowsmith, J and Campbell, C (2000) A comparison of local anaesthetics for venepuncture. *Archives of Disease in Childhood*, 82: 309–10.

Audit Commission (2001) *A Spoonful of Sugar: Medicines management in NHS hospitals*. London: Audit Commission.

British Medical Association (BMA) (2009) Access to Health Records: Guidance for health professionals in the United Kingdom. London: BMA Ethics Department. Available online at www.bma.org.uk (accessed 5 November 2010).

British Medical Association (BMA) and Royal Pharmaceutical Society (RPS) (2009) *Nurse Prescribers' Formulary for Community Practitioners, 2009–11*. London: Pharmaceutical Press.

British Medical Association (BMA), Royal Pharmaceutical Society (RPS), Royal College of Paediatrics and Child Health (RCPCH) and Neonatal and Paediatric Pharmacists Group (2010) *British National Formulary for Children 2010–2011*. London: Pharmaceutical Press. Available online at www.bnfc.org/bnfc (accessed 12 January 2011).

British Thoracic Society (BTS) (1997) Guidelines on current best practice for nebuliser treatment. *Thorax*. 52 (April) (Suppl. 2): 1–106.

British Thoracic Society (BTS)/Scottish Intercollegiate Guidelines Network (SIGN) (2008) *British Guideline on the Management of Asthma*. London: BTS/SIGN.

Burns, DS (2001) The effect of the Bonny method of guided imagery and music on the mood and life quality of cancer patients. *Journal of Music Therapy*, 38 (Spring): 51–65.

Carlton, P, Johnson, I and Cunliffe, C (2009) Factors influencing parents' decisions to choose chiropractic care for their children in the UK. *Clinical Chiropractic*, 12(1): 11–22.

Chappell, K and Newman, C (2004) Potential tenfold drug overdoses on neonatal unit. *Archives of Disease in Childhood – Fetal Neonatal*, 89: 483–4.

Choy, L, Collier, J and Watson, AR (1999) Comparison of lignocaine-prilocaine cream and amethocaine gel for local analgesia before venepuncture in children. *Acta Paediatrica*, 88: 961–44.

Cockayne, N, Duguid, M and Shenfield, GM (2004) Health professionals rarely record history of complementary and alternative medicines. *British Journal Clinical Pharmacology*, 59(2): 254–8.

Conroy, S, North, C and Fox, T, et al. (2008) Educational interventions to reduce prescribing errors. *Archives of Disease in Childhood*, 93: 313–15.

Cook, IF and Murtagh, J (2003) Comparative reactogenecity and parental acceptability of pertussis vaccines administered into the ventrogluteal area and anterolateral thigh in children aged 2, 4, 6 and 18 months old. *Vaccine*, 21(23): 3330–4.

Cook, IF and Murtagh, J (2005) Optimal technique for intramuscular injection of infants and toddlers: a randomised trial. *Medical Journal of Australia*, 183(2): 60–3.

Dailey, RH (1988) Fatality secondary to misuse of TAC solution. *Annals of Emergency Medicine*, 17(2) (February): 159–60.

Department for Education and Skills (DfES) (2003) *National Standards for Under-8s Day-care and Childminding.* Nottingham: DfES Publication Centre.

Department for Education and Skills (DfES) (2005) *Managing Medicines in Schools and Early Years Settings.* London: DfES. Available online at www.teachernet.gov.uk/publications (accessed 27 November 2010).

Department of Health (DH) (1989) *Report of the Advisory Group on Nurse Prescribing* (1st Crown Report). London: Department of Health.

Department of Health (DH) (1996) *Health of the Nation and Young People.* London: Department of Health.

Department of Health (DH) (1999) *Review of the Prescribing, Supply and Administration of Medicines* (2nd Crown Report). London: Department of Health.

Department of Health and Social Security (DHSS) (1986) *Neighbourhood Nursing: A focus for care* (Cumberlege Report). London: DHSS.

Department of Health (DH) (1991) *The Children Act 1989: Guidance and regulations: Volume 6, Children with disabilities.* London: Department of Health.

Department of Health (1997) *The New NHS: Modern, dependable.* London: Department of Health.

Department of Health (DH) (2003) *Getting the Right Start: The National Service Framework for Children, Young People and Maternity Services: Standards for hospital services.* London: The Stationery Office.

Department of Health (DH) (2004a) *National Service Framework for Children, Young People and Maternity Services: Medicines for children and young people.* London: Department of Health.

Department of Health (DH) (2004b) *Publication of Revised Guidelines for Health Professionals on the Provision of Contraceptive Care.* London: Department of Health. Available online at www.ffprhc.org.uk/admin/uploads/under16s.pdf (accessed 5 November 2010).

Department of Health (DH) (2006) *Immunisation Against Infectious Disease – 'The Green Book'.* London: Department of Health.

Department of Health (DH) (2008) *The Child Health Promotion Programme: Pregnancy and the first five years of life.* London: Department of Health.

Department of Health (DH) (2009a) *Birth to Five.* London: Department of Health.

Department of Health (DH) (2009b) *Healthy Lives, Brighter Futures: The strategy for children and young people's health.* London: Department of Health.

Department of Health (DH) (2009c) *Reduce the Risk of Cot Death.* London: Department of Health.

Diggle, L and Deeks, J (2000) Effect of needle length on incidence of local reactions to routine immunisation in infants aged four months: randomised controlled trial. *British Medical Journal*, 321: 931–3.

Diggle, L, Deeks, JJ and Pollard, AJ (2006) Effect of needle size on immunogenicity and reactogenicity of vaccines in infants: randomised controlled trial. *British Medical Journal*, 333: 571–4.

Dyer, C (1999) GMC clears doctors of accidental morphine overdose. *British Medical Journal*, 318(7192) (1 May): 1167.

European Parliament (2006) Regulation (EC) No 1901/2006 of the European Parliament and of the Council of 12 December 2006 on medicinal products for paediatric use and amending Regulation (EEC) No 1768/92, Directive 2001/20/EC, Directive 2001/83/EC and Regulation (EC) No 726/2004. *Official Journal* L378, 27/12/2006, pp1–19.

Ghaleb, MA, Franklin, DB, Barber, N et al. (2006) A systematic review of medication errors in pediatric patients. *Annals of Pharmacotherapy*, 40: 1766–76.

Gillick v *West Norfolk and Wisbech Area Health Authority* (1986) AC 112 at 189 (Lord Scarman).

Gladstone, J (1995) Drug administration errors: a study into the factors underlying the occurrence and reporting of drug errors in a district general hospital. *Journal of Advanced Nursing*, 22: 628–37.

Glatstein, M, Finkelstein, Y and Scolnik, D (2009) Accidental methadone ingestion in an infant: case report and review of the literature. *Pediatric Emergency Care*, 25(2): 109–11.

Gotschall, CS, Morrison, MI and Eichelberger, MR (1998) Prospective, randomized study of the efficacy of Mepitel on children with partial-thickness scalds. *Journal of Burn Care and Rehabilitation*, 19; 279–83.

Health and Safety Commission (2002) *Control of Substances Hazardous to Health Regulations 2002 (as amended 2005)*. Sudbury: HSE Books.

Hemsworth, S (2000) Intramuscular (IM) injection technique. *Paediatric Nursing*, 12(9): 17–20.

House of Commons Select Committee on Health (2004) *The Regulation of Controlled Drugs in the Community*. London: HMSO.

House of Lords (2000) *Complementary and Alternative Medicine: Sixth report from the Select Committee on Science and Technology*. London: The Stationery Office.

Huhtala,V, Lehtonen, L, Heinonen, R and Korvenranta, H (2000) Infant massage compared with crib vibrator in the treatment of colicky infants. *Pediatrics*, 105(6) (June): 84.

John, A and Stevenson, T (1995) A basic guide to the principles of drug therapy. *British Journal of Nursing*, 4: 1194–8.

Jury, L (1996) Hospital drug error may have damaged baby's brain. *The Independent on Sunday*, 18 November. Available online at www.independent.co.uk/news/hospital-drug-error-may-have-damaged-babys-brain-1352974.html (accessed 14 January 2011).

Koren, G, Barzilay, Z and Greenwald, M (1986) Tenfold errors in administration of drug doses: a neglected iatrogenic disease in paediatrics. *Pediatrics*, 77: 848–9.

Lander, J and Fowler-Kerry, S (1993) TENs for children's procedural pain. *Pain*, 52(2) (February): 209–16.

Lawson, RA, Smart, NG and Gudgeon AC, et al. (1995) Evaluation of an amethocaine gel preparation for percutaneous analgesia before venous cannulation in children. *British Journal of Anaesthesia*, 75: 282–5.

Lischner, H, Seligman, SJ, Krammer, A and Parmelee, AH (1961) An outbreak of neonatal deaths among term infants associated with administration of chloramphenicol. *Journal of Pediatrics*, 59(1): 21–34.

MacAuley, DC (2001) Ice therapy: how good is the evidence? *International Journal of Sports Medicine*, 22(5) (July): 379–84.

McKibbon, KA and Walker, CJ (1994) Beyond ACP Journal Club: How to harness Medline for therapy problems. *Annals of Internal Medicine*, 121(1): 125–7.

Medicines and Healthcare products Regulatory Agency (MHRA) (2008) *Devices in Practice: A guide for professionals in health and social care*. London: MHRA.

Miller, J, Cross, M, Gerrett, D and Webb, D (2006) A prioritisation of the most effective interventions for reducing medication errors in UK hospitals as perceived by senior pharmacists. *European Journal of Hospital Pharmacy Science*, 12(2): 23–8.

Moore, ER, Anderson, GC and Bergman, N (2007) Early skin-to-skin contact for mothers and their healthy newborn infants. Cochrane Database of Systematic Reviews, Issue 3. Art. No.: CD003519. DOI: 10.1002/14651858.CD003519.pub2.

Mullin, A, McAuley, RJ, Watts, DJ, Crome, IB and Bloor, RN (2008) Awareness of the need for safe storage of methadone at home is not improved by the use of protocols on recording information giving. *Harm Reduction Journal*, 5: 15. Available online at www.harmreductionjournal.com/content/2/1/9 (accessed 14 January 2011).

National Children's Bureau (NCB) (2008) *Play in Hospital* (Children's Play Information Service Factsheet). London: NCB.

National Collaborating Centre for Women's and Children's Health (2007) *Atopic Eczema in Children: Management of atopic eczema in children from birth up to the age of 12 years*. Commissioned by the National Institute for Health and Clinical Excellence. London: RCOG Press.

National Health Service (NHS) Quality Improvement Scotland (2010) *Home Oxygen Therapy for Children Being Cared For in the Community* (Best Practice Statement). Edinburgh: NHS Scotland. Available online at www.nhs healthquality.org/nhsqis/files/HOTREV_BPS_MAR10.pdf (accessed 14 January 2011).

National Health Service Scotland (NHSS) (2006) *A Multi-Faith Guide for Healthcare Staff*. Edinburgh: NHS Education for Scotland. Available online at www.nes.scot.nhs.uk/publications (accessed 3 December 2010).

National Institute of Health and Clinical Excellence (NICE) (2000) *Asthma (Children under 5): Inhaler devices*. London: NICE. Available online at http://guidance.nice.org.uk/TA10 (accessed 17 October 2010).

National Institute of Health and Clinical Excellence (NICE) (2002) *Asthma (Older Children): Inhaler devices*. London: NICE. Available online at http://guidance.nice.org.uk/TA38 (accessed 17 October 2010).

National Institute for Health and Clinical Excellence (NICE) (2007) *Atopic Eczema in Children (CG57): Management of atopic eczema in children from birth up to the age of 12 years*. London: NICE.

National Patient Safety Agency (NPSA) (2007) *Patient Safety Alert 19: Promoting safer measurement and administration of liquid medicines via oral and enteral routes*. Available online at www.npsa.nhs.uk (accessed 17 October 2007).

NHS Choices (2010) *At What Age Can Children Buy Over the Counter Medicines?* Available online at http://www.nhs.uk/chq/Pages/1009.aspx?CategoryID=73&SubCategoryID=102 (accessed 25 November 2010).

Nursing and Midwifery Council (NMC) (2004) *Guidelines for the Administration of Medicines*. London: NMC.

Nursing and Midwifery Council (NMC) (2006) *Standards of Proficiency for Nurse and Midwife Prescribers*. London: NMC.

Nursing and Midwifery Council (NMC) (2008) *The Code: Standards of conduct, performance and ethics for nurses and midwives*. London: NMC.

Nursing and Midwifery Council (NMC) (2009) *Record Keeping Guidance for Nurses and Midwives*. London: NMC.

Nursing and Midwifery Council (NMC) (2010a) *Standards for Pre-registration Nursing Education*. London: NMC.

Nursing and Midwifery Council (NMC) (2010b) *Standards for Medicines Management*. London: NMC.

Nursing and Midwifery Practice Development Unit (NMPDU) (2002) *Best Practice Statement: Home oxygen therapy for children being cared for in the community*. Edinburgh: NMPDU, NHS Scotland.

Oostema, JA and Ray, DJ (2010) No clear winner among dressings for partial-thickness burns. *Annals of Emergency Medicine*, 56(3): 298–9.

O'Shea, E (1999) Factors contributing to medication errors: a literature review. *Journal of Clinical Nursing*, 8(5):496–504.

Oxford Centre for Evidence-based Medicine (2009) *Levels of Evidence*. Available online at www.cebm.net/index.aspx?o=1025 (accessed 17 November 2010).

Park, EK and Song, M (2004) Communication barriers perceived by older patients and nurses. *International Journal of Nursing Studies*, 42: 159–66.

Pinelli, J and Symington, AJ (2005) Non-nutritive sucking for promoting physiologic stability and nutrition in preterm infants. Cochrane Database of Systematic Reviews, Issue 4. Art. No.: CD001071. DOI: 10.1002/14651858.CD001071.pub2.

Poland, GA, Borrud, A, Jacobson, RM, McDermott, K, Wollan, PC, Brakke, D and Charboneau, JW (1997) Determination of deltoid fat pad thickness: implications for needle length in adult immunization. *Journal of the American Medical Association*, 277: 1709-11.

Resuscitation Council UK (2008) *Emergency Treatment of Anaphylactic Reactions: Guidelines for healthcare providers.* London: Working Group of the Resuscitation Council UK.

Romsing, J, Henneberg, SW and Walther-Larson, S et al. (1999) Tetracaine vs EMLA cream for percutaneous anaesthesia in children. *British Journal of Anaesthesia*, 82: 637–8.

Royal College of Nursing (RCN) (2003) *Complementary Therapies in Nursing, Midwifery and Health Visiting Practice: RCN guidance on integrating complementary therapies into clinical care.* London: RCN.

Royal College of Nursing (RCN) (2009) *Supporting Children and Young People with Diabetes.* London: RCN.

Royal College of Nursing (RCN) (2010) *Standards for the Weighing of Infants, Children and Young People in Acute Healthcare Settings.* London: Royal College of Nursing.

Royal College of Paediatrics and Child Health (RCPCH) (1999) *Medicines for Children.* London: RCPCH.

Royal College of Paediatrics and Child Health (RCPCH) (2000) *Medicines for Children: Information for older children.* London: Royal College of Paediatrics and Child Health/Neonatal and Paediatric Pharmacists Group Standing Committee on Medicines. Available online at www.nes.scot.nhs.uk/pharmacy/paediatrics/Key%20documents/OLDER%20CHILDREN.PDF (accessed 23 November 2010).

Royal College of Paediatrics and Child Health (RCPCH)/Royal College of Nursing (RCN) (2002) *Position Statement on Injection Technique.* London: RCPCH/RCN.

Sackett, DL, Richardson, WS, Rosenberg, WMC and Haynes RB (1997) *Evidence Based Medicine: How to practice and teach evidence based medicine.* London: BMJ Publishing Group.

Sammons, H and Conroy, S (2008) How do we ensure safe prescribing for children? *Archives of Disease in Childhood*, 93: 98–9.

Sandell, JM and Charman, SC (2009) Can age-based estimates of weight be safely used when resuscitating children? *Emergency Medicine Journal*, 26: 43–7.

Sharkey, I, Boddy, AV, Wallace, H, Mycroft, J, Hollis, R and Picton, S (2001) Body surface area estimation in children using weight alone: application in paediatric oncology. *British Journal of Cancer*, 85(1): 23–8.

Soanes, N (2000) Injection site safety. *Nursing Standard*, 14(25): 55.

Stubenrauch, JM (2007) Striving for distraction: Two nurses are honored for research on an innovative approach to pain management. *American Journal of Nursing*, 107(3): 94–5.

Tan, E, Cranswick, NE and Rayner, CR et al. (2003) Dosing information for paediatric patients: are they really 'therapeutic orphans'? *Medical Journal of Australia*, 179: 195–8.

United Nations General Assembly (1989) *Conventions on the Rights of the Child.* New York: United Nations.

Van Kam, HJM, Egberts, ACG and Rijnvos, WPM et al. (1997) Tetracaine versus lidocaine-prilocaine for preventing venepuncture-induced pain in children. *American Journal of Health-System Pharmacy*, 54: 388–92.

Walsh, KE, Kaushal, R and Chessare, JB (2005) How to avoid paediatric medication errors: a user's guide to the literature. *Archives of Disease in Childhood*, 90: 698–702.

Wasiak, J, Cleland, H and Campbell, F (2008) Dressings for superficial and partial-thickness burns. *Cochrane Database Systematic Review*, 4: CD002106. DOI: 10.1002/14651858.CD002106.pub3.

World Health Organization (WHO) (2004) *Immunization in Practice: A guide for health workers.* Geneva: WHO.

Workman, B (1999) Safe injection techniques. *Nursing Standard*, 13(39): 47–53.

Zaybak, A, Gunes, UY, Tamsel, S, Khorshid, L and Eser, I (2007) Does obesity prevent the needle from reaching muscle in intramuscular injections? *Journal of Advanced Nursing*, 58(6): 552–6.

Zuckerman, JN (2000) The importance of injecting vaccine into muscle. *British Medical Journal*, 321: 1237–8.

Index